TAKE CONTROL OF YOUR **WEIGHT**

TAKE CONTROL
OF YOUR
WEIGHT

Dr. Jonas's
Program for Success

STEVEN JONAS, M.D.

and the Editors of
Consumer Reports Books

CONSUMER REPORTS BOOKS

A Division of Consumers Union

Yonkers, New York

For Adrienne

Copyright © 1993 by Steven Jonas

Published by Consumers Union of United States, Inc., Yonkers, New York 10703.

Library of Congress Cataloging-in-Publication Data

Jonas, Steven.
    Take control of your weight : Dr. Jonas's program for success /
Steven Jonas, and the editors of Consumer Reports Books.
        p.   cm.
    Includes bibliographical references and index.
    ISBN 0-89043-549-9 — ISBN 0-89043-535-9 (H).
    1. Reducing.   I. Consumer Reports Books.   II. Title.
    RM222.2.J616   1993
    613.2'5—dc20   92-41124
                                                      CIP

Stretching exercises on pages 137–39 from *Get in Shape, Stay in Shape* by F. Skip Latella, Winifred
Conkling, and the Editors of Consumer Reports Books. Copyright © 1989 by F. Skip Latella and
Consumers Union. Reprinted by permission of Consumers Union.

"Fat Grams per Serving" on pages 74–8 from *Food Values of Portions Commonly Used*, 14th ed., by
Janet A. T. Pennington and Helen Nichols Church. Copyright © 1980, 1985 by Janet A. T.
Pennington, Ph.D., R.D., and Helen Nichols Church, B.S. Reprinted by permission of HarperCollins
Publishers.

Design by Joy Taylor
First printing, May 1993
This book is printed on recycled paper. ✪
Manufactured in the United States of America

Take Control of Your Weight is a Consumer Reports Book published by Consumers Union, the
nonprofit organization that publishes *Consumer Reports*, the monthly magazine of test reports,
product Ratings, and buying guidance. Established in 1936, Consumers Union is chartered under the
Not-For-Profit Corporation Law of the State of New York. The purposes of Consumers Union, as
stated in its charter, are to provide consumers with information and counsel on consumer goods and
services, to give information on all matters relating to the expenditure of the family income, and to
initiate and to cooperate with individual and group efforts seeking to create and maintain decent
living standards.

    Consumers Union derives its income solely from the sale of *Consumer Reports* and other
publications. In addition, expenses of occasional public service efforts may be met, in part, by
nonrestrictive, noncommercial contributions, grants, and fees. Consumers Union accepts no
advertising or product samples and is not beholden in any way to any commercial interest. Its
Ratings and reports are solely for the use of the readers of its publications. Neither the Ratings, nor
the reports, nor any Consumers Union publication, including this book, may be used in advertising
or for any commercial purpose. Consumers Union will take all steps open to it to prevent such uses
of its material, its name, or the name of *Consumer Reports*.

ACKNOWLEDGMENTS

THANKS to my agent, Harvey Klinger, for having faith in me and this book. It would not have seen the light of day without him.

At Consumer Reports Books, my appreciation and thanks goes to Sarah Uman for her understanding and endorsement of this new concept in weight loss, and for her patience and hard work in seeing this project through. Thanks also to Darlene Bledsoe for a thoughtful and perceptive job of line editing that enriched the final product, and Julie Henderson, who skillfully saw this manuscript through the production stages.

It was during my work on two earlier books, *PaceWalking: The Balanced Way to Aerobic Health* (coauthored by Peter Radetsky) and *The "I-Don't-Eat (but-I-Can't-Lose)" Weight-Loss Program* (coauthored by Virginia Aronson, R.D., M.S.), that I did some of the original thinking and writing that eventually led to the creation of this book. I learned a great deal about food and nutrition from Ms. Aronson, who is both a well-known nutritionist and an accomplished writer. I thank her very much for sharing her knowledge so freely. That knowledge and learning provided me with a solid foundation for the concepts expressed in this book. Many thanks to Peter Radetsky for what he showed me about writing.

I wish to thank the following persons for providing helpful suggestions, encouragement, and information during the development of this book: Sharon Bortz, Ph.D.; Kelly Brownell, Ph.D.; Karen Donato, M.A., Ph.D.; Jean-Pierre Flatt, Ph.D.; David Garner, Ph.D.; Janey Milstead; Michael Perri, Ph.D.; Barbara Rimer, Ph.D.; Judith Stern, Ph.D.; Adrienne Weiss, M.S.W.; and David Williamson, Ph.D.

CONTENTS

PREFACE
A Personal View

AUTHORS of books on how to lose weight come from a variety of disciplines and backgrounds. They include nutritionists, clinical physicians, psychologists, health educators, and exercise specialists. Some are journalists or writers who either team up with a health science professional or learn about weight loss independently. A few authors are charlatans who, without regard for scientific facts and healthy eating, dream up some weight-loss gimmick that they then publish, hoping to appear on TV talk shows and sell a million copies.

I am among the authors who come from a public health background, with knowledge of nutritional principles and experience in problem identification, causal analysis, and program planning. This book presents the weight/fat-loss program that I developed based on my professional experience analyzing the problem as a public health physician, and on my personal experience as well.

How It All Began

The idea of controlling my weight had its genesis many years ago. In the course of my research in health policy, I wrote a book on medical education reform entitled *Medical Mystery: The Training of Doctors in the United States.** I called for major changes in medical education, proposing that its primary focus on disease be redirected, first to health, second to disease. That book led me to work as a consultant on medical education and preventive medicine at the Texas College of Osteopathic Medicine (TCOM) in Fort Worth, in the spring of 1980.

Many people at Texas College took the idea of health and fitness very seri-

---

*Steven Jonas, *Medical Mystery: The Training of Doctors in the United States* (New York: W. W. Norton, 1978).

ously. When I started working there, most of my own health risk factors were fairly low. Still, I was somewhat overweight (about 10 percent over the upper limit of normal for my height and build), and though I did not know it at the time, I was considerably over*fat* (at 26 percent body weight).

I was forced to focus on the fact that I didn't exercise, while so many of my students and colleagues obviously did. I was the "expert" on disease prevention, but soon realized that in order to be effective, I must practice what I preached. But because I was dealing with only *external* pressures to become a regular exerciser—not effective motivators of behavioral change—nothing happened.

In fact, nothing happened for about six months. Then one day I walked up a ramp at a convention center in Detroit and was huffing and puffing by the time I got to the top. That's it, I said to myself. I've had enough of this being-out-of-shape business. When I get home I'm going to begin exercising.

I now wanted to exercise for *me,* and recognized that I had to exercise for *me,* not for anyone else.

First Steps: Overcoming Fear of Failure

Although I had decided to pursue physical fitness, I really had no background or training in an exercise program. I had been a virtual nonathlete all my life and had never thought of myself as anything else. Well, you can run, I said to myself. Running is a sport that requires no physical skill. You'll just go slowly.

While I didn't think about it at the time, I now wonder if my previous failure to exercise was partially because of my own nonathletic self-image. Was I living in fear of failing at an activity that is natural to almost every living creature? If fear was part of it, and I believe it was, the desire to become fit finally overcame that fear. If I were going to achieve something that had suddenly become very important to me, I would have to risk failure.

From Runner to Triathlete

I began working out on the local high school track, going slowly and gradually building up endurance. My first goal was to run for 20 minutes without stopping. That personal approach to exercise became the model that I now recommend to everyone who is just starting out.

By the end of that first winter, I had achieved my original goals, and I had set new ones. At the end of the year, having read about the advantages of doing more than one aerobic sport, I bought my first 10-speed bike. With the coming of spring, I set a new running goal: to do a 5-mile road race. I was becoming a real athlete, exploring my boundaries. I now call the process *exploring limits, recognizing limitations.*

I ran that 5-mile race without once walking or stopping. Then I entered a 10-k (10 kilometers, 6.2 miles) race. One thing led to another: a 20-mile road race, a marathon, and in between, my first multisport race, the Mighty Hamptons Triathlon, held in Sag Harbor, New York, in 1983. Eventually I did an ironman distance triathlon (2.4-mile swim, 112-mile bike, 26.2-mile [marathon] run), albeit slowly (16 hours and 42 minutes the first time). Recognizing my limitations, I found that if I stayed within certain boundaries in terms of speed, I could swim, bike, and run for a very long time and distance. I lost fat, gained muscle, became fit, and discovered the athlete within me.

Discovering Your Strengths

Not everyone has to set new goals for distance, speed, and endurance to stay involved in an exercise program. Just because I did it this way, and found it so helpful in keeping motivated, doesn't mean that you have to do it this way. Whatever works for *you,* whatever keeps *you* going, is good.

Nor is it necessary for you to become an athlete or a racer. I am saying, though, look inside yourself. You may find, as I did, that you have the strength to lose permanently the 30 extra pounds of fat your body has been quietly storing for the past 10 years, protecting itself against the famine that will never come. Sometimes just going to the gym three times a week to do Nautilus, when you always thought you didn't belong there with all those muscular bodies, is an accomplishment. You can build muscle and lose fat, too. Or you may find the motivation and commitment to fastwalk a five-kilometer road race, or do a four-hour triathlon. If you are like most of us, you'll find inside yourself hidden treasures of strength and personal control.

Of course, it wasn't only the regular exercise that made me a different person. I changed my eating habits, too.

Altering Eating Patterns

Many dietary plans require that you completely change your food intake within eight, six, or even four weeks. I didn't do it that way, and I don't expect you to do it either. Such a radical approach rarely works anyway. The changes in my own eating habits started several years before I began exercising regularly. At that time, I was concerned chiefly about reducing my consumption of fat, so I gradually eliminated certain foods from my diet.

Bacon. For example, I decided to stop eating bacon, a very high-fat food. I still eat it when dining out every once in a while. I just don't serve it at home.

Beef. I also ate a lot of red meat—hamburger, steak, pot roast, roast beef—often four to five times a week. This change was very gradual—it took me over a year to cut back on the red meats. I now eat only one or two meals each week that include beef, pork, or lamb. As well as decreasing frequency, I also gradually decreased the portion size.

At first, I substituted chicken, turkey, or fish for the beef. Now, over the course of a year, I average two to three dinners each week totally without meat. I started eating meatless meals once a week, then twice, and so on. I found that I really liked this regimen, that it made me feel better. And doing it on a gradual basis made the transition a lot easier.

Chocolate. I was a true chocoholic, eating lots of chocolate candy and cake, loving my hot fudge on ice cream. (The main problem with chocolate, by the way, is the fat, not the sugar.) So I started by not buying a package of peanut chews every time I went to the movies, refraining from eating a chocolate bar or two every time I took an airplane flight, and not keeping chocolate candy in the house. Again, I reduced my chocolate intake bit by chocolate bit. Now I consume very little. When I do eat chocolate, I thoroughly enjoy it, but I don't feel the need to eat much at one time. I know that the next morning I will have an engorged feeling in my throat if I overdo it. My body's reaction now helps keep my chocolate fat intake down.

Ice cream. I love ice cream, so this was a toughie. Hot-fudge sundaes were a favorite. My reduction in chocolate consumption and the development of the negative reaction to chocolate helped me to reduce my ice-cream consumption as well. Now, even when I have an occasional sundae, it's almost always a fruit sundae, not hot fudge. (Fruit toppings contain sugar and calories, but little or no fat.)

I often have sherbet with fruit, and have developed a taste for frozen low- or nonfat yogurt. As a substitute for ice cream, I have increased my fruit intake: fresh, canned, or frozen. I have learned to enjoy the different flavors and natural sugars.

Milk. I drink a fair amount of milk. I always have. Years ago, you could buy only whole milk and skim milk. Inveterate milk-drinkers found it hard to switch from whole to skim, since skim seemed to have neither body nor flavor. But now you can get milk with 2 percent fat or 1 percent fat. Make the change gradually, as I did, going from whole to 2 percent to 1 percent and all the way down to skim, if you prefer. Actually, I use mainly 1 percent fat, and skim occasionally. Whole milk now tends to give me that overfull, too-much-fat feeling.

Cookies. High-fat cookies (most cookies) vanished from my home and diet. I found that if I had them in the house, I would eat them. It's interesting that I got few complaints from my kids on this; as my diet was changing, so was theirs. They were also becoming less interested in fatty foods. We still occasionally have some low-fat cookies around, like fig newtons, oatmeal (check the label to make sure that any added fats are unsaturated, not palm or coconut), and gingersnaps. I have also developed a taste for cinnamon graham crackers.

Cake. I used to eat a lot of cake, especially chocolate cake. I eat cake rarely now, chocolate cake almost never. I'm sure that you can see the pattern: Changing your eating of one kind of fatty food will influence your eating of another. Now for a sweet dessert I almost always have a piece of fruit pie. This dessert may be high in calories because of the sugar, but most of the fat in fruit pies, especially homemade ones, is found in the crusts, and not in the fillings.

Chicken. Is chicken a source of fat? Yes, indeed. The fat lies in and under the skin. This was another difficult change for me. I enjoy eating chicken, but I love the skin, fried or broiled. Then I took a good look at the fat that can pour out of a fast-food, deep-fried chicken breast. I still eat it occasionally, but I don't fool myself that it's providing a low-fat meal. And I order smaller portions, to avoid that post-fatty-food feeling. Of course the fast-food, no-coating grilled chicken sandwiches, with no sauce or mayo, do provide a good low-fat meal.

At home, I eat broiled skinless chicken breasts and use a variety of flavorful seasonings to enhance the taste. And I still broil a rack of drumsticks when the mood strikes me, cooking them well to eliminate as much of the fat as possible.

Cheese. Cheese was one of my favorite foods, especially the hard, strongly flavored varieties that are high in saturated fat. I used to eat on average at least a quarter of a pound a day, some in the morning for breakfast, and some as a late-night snack. Actually, I stuck with cheese long after I reduced other fats in my diet. I put up with the bloated feeling in the morning because of the enjoyment that the texture and flavor of cheese gave me at night.

But one day I decided that I no longer wanted to experience the next-morning, cheese-the-night-before horrors. As a side benefit, I would be further reducing my fat intake. So eight years after we stopped buying bacon, we stopped buying cheese. Once again I found that I didn't miss it. I was ready in my mind and in my body to give up this food. Now I rarely eat cheese, and it seldom finds its way into our refrigerator, usually only when my son demands it.

Final Thoughts

As you can see, I didn't rush the changes; I made them only when and if I felt that I could make them. So don't rush to throw out the cheese or cookies. There is no hurry. Haste can frequently lead to failure.

Since you are reading this book, you have probably been overweight/overfat and/or out of shape for many years. You can't reverse overnight, or even in two weeks, what those years have done to your body. But if you take control, set up a regular schedule of exercise, and begin to change your eating habits gradually, you will feel changes in your head in a week or two, and see changes in your body in a month or so. If you stick with it, your appearance will probably change noticeably in three months and markedly in six. And the chances are very great that these alterations will stay with you for the rest of your life.

In summary, anyone who wants to lose weight permanently should follow these five steps to success:

- Take control of your life and body
- Respond only to internal motivation
- Set clear and reasonable goals
- Explore your limits while recognizing your limitations
- Make changes gradually

It is no accident that these steps form the basic principles of the Take Control of Your Weight Program outlined in this book.

Scientific Basis of This Book

The theory and practice of this book are based on proven metabolic, nutritional, and epidemiological scientific evidence. For example, there is little scientific controversy over the concept that (1) at any one time body weight is the product of something more than simply calories in/calories out, or (2) a combination of low-fat eating and exercise is the healthy approach to losing weight, and over time will result in weight loss in a significant number of people.

However, the reader should be aware that there is debate over certain components of the weight-loss theory in this book. For example, not every nutritional scientist agrees that the evidence is clear that the starvation response necessarily leads to a reduction in the resting metabolic rate. Nor do all nutritional scientists agree that exercise will necessarily raise the resting metabolic rate of all persons who try it.

The truth is that significant gaps exist in our knowledge of both the metabolism and the epidemiology of weight gain/weight loss, especially the epidemiology. Much research remains to be done; however, it is quite clear that low-fat eating and regular exercise are the healthy, safe ways to approach individual nutrition and metabolism, and indeed are the only fully healthy methods of weight reduction. Even if you are in an unusual situation (e.g., suffering from a form of massive obesity or from some underlying disease that affects your metabolism in an obscure way), or if you are one of those people who cannot lose at least some weight by eating a low-fat diet and regularly exercising, you will not harm yourself by cutting your fat intake and beginning some form of regular exercise. And you will be decreasing your risk for diseases and negative physical conditions that can result from a high-fat diet.

Health-care professionals currently have two choices in proposing approaches to weight losss. We can wait for all the scientific evidence, both metabolic and epidemiological, to come in before making any proposals. Or, we can make recommendations based on the weight of current scientific evidence and theory, as we see and understand it. If we choose the latter approach, we can also strive to make certain that we have made no harmful recommendations, even if future studies should prove some aspect of the theory wrong. In the process, we can attempt to create a weight-loss approach and program that has a good chance of working successfully for many of the people who try it. That is what I have chosen to do.

TAKE CONTROL OF YOUR **WEIGHT**

INTRODUCTION

Central Premises of the
Take Control of Your Weight Program

Most authorities accept that many millions of Americans are overweight. The public hardly takes this situation lightly. At one time or another, through one diet plan or another, most Americans concerned about their weight have tried to slim down. In fact, dieting Americans may already have lost hundreds of millions of pounds, surely a world record. Unfortunately, the total amount of weight regained may be only slightly less than was lost, and according to some estimates even more.

While we do not have exact figures on how successful Americans are in keeping off their lost pounds, we do know that the success rate is rather low for those in organized programs (whether commercial or hospital-based), in the 5 to 10 percent range. On the other hand, those who have lost weight on their own may have a much higher success rate.

Those who see themselves through a weight-loss process without direct outside supervision or regular support may also be successful in permanently keeping off at least some significant portion of the lost weight. So the fact that you have come to this book prepared to do something about your weight, on your own, makes your prospects for long-range success better than you might have assumed when you first started to think about attempting a weight-loss program.

One reason for this difference in success rates may be that an important predictor of successful weight loss is the extent to which a person is prepared to take personal control, rather than surrender that control to another person or an impersonal program. For the purposes of this book, we define taking control as:

> Deciding to assume guidance of an authority over your body and
>   behavior
> Equipping yourself with the tools necessary for weight loss
> Establishing a realistic goal
> Assuming personal responsibility for the results

To the extent we can know the truth in an area in which so little scientific research has been done, it appears that even if we were to set aside the question of personal control, all weight-loss programs would still not be alike. At one time the traditional wisdom was that losing weight involved little more than eating fewer calories than we burned.*

Now we know that things are not that simple. For example, the source of the calories—fat, protein, or carbohydrates—is very important, as well as whether or not the nutrients in your diet are balanced enough to give you the energy to manage your life constructively. We shall go into greater detail about a properly balanced diet later on, but for now it is enough to stress that nutritionally sound eating habits can make a significant contribution to your success, as well as ensuring that you do not harm yourself during your weight-loss program.

One of the premises of the Take Control of Your Weight Program is that successful, comfortable, permanent, and healthy weight loss requires taking control of those factors that can lead to overweight in general, and then focusing on those particular patterns that are most responsible for your own overweight.

The three most common contributions to overweight are eating, lack of physical activity, and a poor self-image.

Eating. In most cases, though not all, being overweight involves having poor eating habits. Not all overweight people are overeaters—in fact it may well be that many are undereaters—but most have some kind of eating problem that must be dealt with in order to lose weight successfully. (One small-scale study did find, in a nonrandom sampling, that certain overweight people

---

*The body really doesn't burn calories. Calories are a measure of energy available in certain nutrients and as such cannot themselves be burned. But because this is such a convenient way to imagine the process by which the carbohydrates, proteins, and fats are converted into energy, rather than stored as fat, we shall take some poetic license in this book and refer to burning calories.

who think they are undereating are not, in fact, actually doing so. Still, there is no way to know from the study whether this would be true of many other "undereating," overweight individuals who are attempting to lose weight.)

However, your eating pattern does not exist in a vacuum. Surrounding it are food choices, and behind food choices are food shopping and food preparation. This book will show you how to empower yourself to take control of all these food-related activities.

Lack of physical activity. The sedentary life-style of many Americans contributes both to weight gain and to the failure of many to lose weight and keep it off. Although regular exercise is not an absolute essential for all successful weight loss, it is certainly a most valuable facilitator. As difficult as it can be to embark on a regular exercise program, failing to do so in many cases dooms your attempts to control your weight to almost endless frustration and despair. The information in this book is not designed to turn you into a world-class athlete. Rather, it will show you how to take control of your physical activity in a happy, healthy way, a way that suits you just as you are.

Poor self-image. Mental image is important in influencing the size and shape of your body, as well as your overall appearance. As part of an attempt to help you take control of those factors that cause you to expect success or failure in dealing with weight loss, this book will help you understand some of the internal and external causes that determine how you think about yourself. This book will also help you learn to mobilize your mental resources to support your efforts to take control of your weight.

The Pathfinder Approach

Another premise of this book is that you must understand how and why you gained the extra weight if you wish to lose the weight and keep it off permanently. Contrary to the traditional way of looking at weight maintenance, it is quite likely that there is not just one pathway to becoming overweight. We now know with some authority that for many people weight gain is more complex than simply taking in too many calories and expending too few.

It seems reasonable to assume that if there is more than one pathway up to a higher weight, there must be more than one pathway back down to a lower weight. A guiding principle of the Take Control of Your Weight Program is that in most cases successful weight loss is greatly aided by choosing the pathway back down that is designed to deal with the one you took up to your present weight. We call the method based on this principle the *Pathfinder Approach*.

You and Dieting for Weight Loss

If you are reading this book, chances are that you have tried to lose weight in the past and were less than satisfied with the results over time. In most of your past attempts, you probably lost weight at the outset. But, like many other people, you may have gradually regained the weight. Possibly, you are now even heavier than you were before you began dieting. That experience is somewhat common and is illustrated in the old story of the person who runs into a close friend after many years apart: "How did you get so heavy?" asks the first person tactlessly. "Constant dieting," replies the friend with a shrug. "How else?"

You may have blamed yourself for the failure of your attempts to lose weight and maintain that weight loss. You may believe that you snatched defeat from the jaws of victory because you lost willpower, that you might have succeeded if only you could have found some way to sustain your willpower for a little longer. The truth is that if you were able to lose weight in the past but soon gained it back you were most likely wrong to blame yourself. In many cases of short-term success/long-term failure the trouble lies not with you or your lack of willpower, but instead with the weight-loss plans you used, many of which are poorly designed and provide virtually no prospects for success.

Diet Plans That Don't Work

Among weight-loss plans that don't work are those based solely or predominantly on severely limiting caloric intake whether by following strict menus or using behavioral techniques (small bites, smaller portions). These plans have no demonstrated records of success in helping people achieve and maintain weight loss, and indeed are often shown to have been counterproductive. One of the hidden consequences of severe diets is that such sudden and dramatic decreases in the number of calories available for necessary body functions can panic your body, causing it to conserve energy resources stored in body fat by slowing down your resting metabolic rate (RMR). Thus, such plans often contribute directly to regaining your lost weight. As a consequence, trying to get back on the right path by cutting calories further won't accomplish much, and could do more harm.

Another kind of diet plan is organized in two stages. The idea is that you will be able to stay with an initially severe approach to weight loss, because you know that once you reach a certain plateau you will be on a more forgiving maintenance diet. However, even if you are able to stay on the first-stage diet, doing so would be unhealthy, because of the depression of the RMR. But as an additional problem, when you move from the first stage to the second you must suddenly learn a new pattern of eating, increasing the risk that you will soon be back to those pre-diet patterns your body knows best of all.

Beyond the problems related to how your body works are others related to the workings of your mind. Few diets actively involve the dieter in designing and carrying out the program. Most focus on *what,* according to the designers, you *should* eat. You are not in control; the diet is. In effect, you are told, "Stop eating whatever foods you are eating, right now, and start eating these other foods, right now. If you do as you are told, you'll lose weight."

At the point where you should be assuming greater control over your life, you are told you have no choices, that the program is run by experts and if you can't make it, you—not the program—are the failure. You become a foot soldier in someone else's march to success, no longer in control of your own destiny. In many of these diets there is no recognition that different people eat differently; no appreciation of the effectiveness and relative ease of gradual, rather than all-at-once change; no understanding of what is needed in terms of taking control to make the long-term changes in eating patterns that are now recognized as the key to weight-loss maintenance.

Although you were learning by hard experience that many diets don't work, you didn't give up wanting to lose weight. There is a good chance that even after one, two, or three failures, you tried yet another diet that, while wearing a different guise, really aimed at the same thing: simple calorie restriction, achieved by your eating exactly what you were told to eat. And that, as you will see, is probably a major factor in many weight-control failures.

The Take Control Philosophy of Weight Loss

If you are going to be able to use the Take Control of Your Weight Program to lose weight or, at a minimum, trade in some of your excess body fat for muscle, we must be on the same wavelength when it comes to what can be called "the philosophy of weight loss." In the first instance, we must agree, and indeed you must be convinced, that losing weight is a good idea for you right now. This is not quite the same as the related issue of whether or not it is possible for more than a very small proportion of overweight people to lose weight, an issue we'll return to in just a moment.

Is Overweight Okay?

Because the Take Control of Your Weight philosophy is predicated on your taking control of your life, another of its premises is that being overweight, and staying that way, is okay. That is, it's okay if that's where you really want to be. The Take Control view agrees that there is much too much cultural emphasis on thinness, especially among women.

The Take Control philosophy agrees that it's okay to weigh more than medical charts say you should, provided that you have carefully considered the risks and benefits of being overweight and have made your own decision to face these risks and accept them (see Appendix A). Unfortunately, many people accept the risks of being overweight because they believe there is nothing they can do about their weight. However, the Take Control program assumes that it is possible for overweight people to lose weight and keep it off. Don't confuse the position "It's okay to be overweight," which is based on a value judgment, with the position that it's hopeless to try to lose weight because of metabolic factors. The first position, we would agree, is a defensible social philosophy. The second doesn't seem to be supported either by metabolic science or by evidence on the epidemiology of obesity.

This is not to say that there is no genetic trigger for obesity, for genetics surely has some influence on body size and shape. But conceding this does not require the next leap in logic—that we are all born to attain a predetermined weight. Many of us, our individual genetic makeup to the contrary, have the power to reduce or increase our weight to a level with which we are more comfortable. To use an analogy, people who have family histories of heart disease can, by reducing all controllable factors, live longer and healthier lives than others who have no history of heart disease but who smoke, consume foods high in saturated fats, and avoid all exercise.

If you prefer to lose weight but continue to doubt that people can alter their weights permanently, you should consider the evidence presented in chapters 1 and 3, both on its terms and in light of your experience, before embarking on the Take Control program. Then, take control! Evaluate what you have read. Make up your mind. Ask yourself if you really think it can work. Can it work for you? We are persuaded by the evidence that you will have a good chance of achieving success, but more important, you must be convinced. If you are, then you should get going.

Successful Weight Loss

Permanence

At one time people described their dieting success in terms of how many pounds they had lost. Now we know better. Today almost everyone defines success not just by how much weight was lost, but also by whether or not the weight has stayed off over time. Another measure of success is whether or not a person is able to maintain a desirable weight without permanently remaining on a calorie-restricted diet.

These current standards of success cannot be achieved just by reducing caloric intake for some finite period. Rather, you must change the way you eat, and often how you expend energy. In order to be of more than transient value, a weight-loss program must help you make *permanent* changes in your eating habits and patterns of physical activity. It must make normal, healthy eating part of your life from the very beginning of the program.

The Take Control of Your Weight Program teaches that learning to eat a healthy, satisfying diet is a first goal, not something you start to think about only after you've reached your weight-loss goal.

Doing It on Your Own

As we have pointed out, the limited research available on weight loss shows that most people who have success losing weight and keeping it off do so on their own, rather than in organized programs (see chapter 2). According to one provocative study, the long-term success rate in do-it-yourself weight loss may be as high as 60 percent. Perhaps many of these people have undertaken the kind of personal, take-control-of-your-life journey featured in our program. They probably did not use the usual quick-weight-loss diet books, but personally collected the information needed to change their own eating and exercise practices, and were prepared to act as their own coaches in putting a sensible plan into action.

Your Role in Weight Loss

If you say you want to lose weight, you should be believed. But to achieve weight loss you may need help, the right kind of help. First and most important, you need not only reliable information in which you can have confidence, but also some understanding of the most important principles involved. You also need a program that is tailored to you and meets your needs, a program that is nutritionally sound and fits your eating habits and general life-style. Given the right tools, you can do the job.

Where do you find such a program? Who will design it for you? Who will show you how to carry it out? In most cases, *you* are the best designer and implementer of a program that will work particularly well for *you*. You know what and how much you eat. You probably have some idea of how you should eat, both for good health and for reducing your weight to a comfortable level and keeping it there. And if exercise is an essential part of your successful weight-loss regimen, as it is for most people, you know or can easily determine which kinds of exercise can fit into your activities without much difficulty, and which kinds will work for you both physically and mentally.

This book presents the kinds of information you need to put together a program that will work for you. It will provide you with the details you need to convert your general understanding into a healthy program of food shopping, cooking, and eating. It will show you how to develop a program of regular exercise that suits you. This book will also demonstrate why taking control is one of the cornerstones of success. Most important, the Take Control of Your Weight Program is based on well-understood and sound scientific, nutritional, and metabolic principles you can trust to protect your health while you move toward your goal. Because you will not only design the details of your program yourself but also supervise their implementation, you have an especially good chance of success.

Weight Gain and Weight Loss in the United States

What Is Overweight?

Many of us are familiar with tables of "normal" weights. Table I.1 is from the 1990 edition of *Dietary Guidelines for Americans,* published by the U.S. Department of Agriculture/U.S. Department of Health and Human Services. Such tables can be helpful, but do they give you all the information you need? Let's say you are a 31-year-old female who is 5 feet 8 inches tall and weighs 155 pounds. Are you overweight? Well, the table notes say that the higher weight in the range given for your age and height (125 to 164 pounds) is for males; therefore, strictly speaking, you are overweight since you are over the table's limits. But is the table's information enough to tell you that you are overweight, and in fact so much so that you should lose weight? Not at all.

Suppose you are a well-conditioned volleyball player who competes regularly, and whose body-fat proportion is 15 percent, two percentage points below that of the range for the average woman (see Table I.2). Although technically you are overweight, you certainly don't need to lose weight. In fact, if you wish to increase your upper-body strength in order to improve your game, you may well need to gain weight, in the form of muscle, not lose it. The same reasoning would apply to a 28-year-old, 6-foot-tall, 205-pound male who has a body-fat percentage of 7 and is a strong safety in the National Football League.

TABLE I.1 *Suggested Weights for Adults*

| Height[1] | Weight in Pounds[2] | |
	19 to 34 Years	35 Years and Over
5'0"	[3]97–128	108–138
5'1"	101–132	111–143
5'2"	104–137	115–148
5'3"	107–141	119–152
5'4"	111–146	122–157
5'5"	114–150	126–162
5'6"	118–155	130–167
5'7"	121–160	134–172
5'8"	125–164	138–178
5'9"	129–169	142–183
5'10"	132–174	146–188
5'11"	136–179	151–194
6'0"	140–184	155–199
6'1"	144–189	159–205
6'2"	148–195	164–210
6'3"	152–200	168–216
6'4"	156–205	173–222
6'5"	160–211	177–228
6'6"	164–216	182–234

Source: U.S. Department of Agriculture/U.S. Department of Health and Human Services, *Dietary Guidelines for Americans,* 3d ed. (Washington, D.C.: Government Printing Office, 1990), 9.
[1]Without shoes.
[2]Without clothes.
[3]The higher weights in the ranges generally apply to men, who tend to have more muscle and bone; the lower weights more often apply to women, who have less muscle and bone.

So, we are not concerned solely with weight. We are also concerned with the configuration of the weight.

What Is Obesity?

Note that Table I.2 defines obesity on the basis of body fat, not overall weight, a relatively new approach. Body weight is comprised primarily of fat, muscle,

TABLE I.2 *Ranges of Body-Fat Percentage*

	Females Percentage Body Fat	Males Percentage Body Fat
Athletes	less than 10	less than 17
Lean	10–15	17–22
Normal	15–18	22–25
Above average	18–20	25–29
Overfat	20–25	29–35
Obese	25 plus	35 plus

and bone. Nerves, brain, skin, connective tissue (e.g., the sheaths that cover muscles), and body fluids such as blood make up the bulk of the remaining weight. When we talk about losing weight, we should really focus on losing extra body fat, not weight. This important distinction must be understood by anyone considering any weight-loss program, because it is quite unhealthy to achieve weight loss through a reduction in overall body mass, which is precisely what happens in many straight calorie-reduction programs.

Many people use the terms *overweight* and *obesity* interchangeably. Although such loose usage does little harm in daily conversation, health-care practitioners give the terms discrete meanings. Most often, obesity is now defined as "a state of having too much body fat," not as carrying too much weight. In most cases of obesity, the person is also overweight. However, within the current definition of obesity, a person can be obese without being overweight if he or she is carrying too high a percentage of body fat, despite the fact that overall body weight may be within the limits described in Table I.1.

Loss of fat will benefit the person of normal weight whose percentage of body fat is too high as well as the overweight person, who will lose weight as well as fat. Depending upon how much exercise is done, the person of normal weight may actually gain weight by adding muscle—by volume heavier than fat—as pounds of fat are lost. Despite the added weight, the person will be healthier and probably look better.

If *obese* is the more technically correct term, you might ask why we don't use it instead of *overweight*. The reason is that many people think *obese* has a more unpleasant, pejorative sound than *overweight*. Although *overweight* is the word primarily used throughout this book, think of it as meaning excess weight in the form of extra fat, the most common form of obesity.

Today some scientists do define obesity in the more traditional way, by excess overall weight. This system defines mild obesity as being between 20 and 40 percent above the upper end of the normal range for your height and weight (see Table I.1), moderate as 41 to 100 percent overweight, and severe (sometimes called morbid obesity) as more than 100 percent overweight.

How to Use This Book

Chapter 1 is devoted primarily to metabolism, and chapter 2 discusses the principles of motivation, including why and how you can put yourself into action in any venture and how to persevere as you encounter difficulties. Chapter 3 focuses on the common problems of eating and exercising faced by most potential dieters, and on the ways that gradual change is central to the process of altering both how you eat and how you expend energy.

The Take Control of Your Weight Program is presented in chapters 4 through 8. The program specifies the building blocks for eating and exercising you will need to include in your own weight-loss program. Instead of engaging you with menus and calorie counting, the program presents detailed food tables and eating pattern logs to help you identify the foods and eating patterns that can cause weight gain. Then you are introduced to *food substitution,* the program's principal tool for helping you change your eating habits.

You will begin to deal with your inconsistent and unhealthy eating patterns. Taking simple, small steps one at a time, and choosing healthier foods from the extensive lists we provide, help you to reduce *gradually* the amounts of certain foods that cause weight gain (e.g., red meat, chocolate, cakes, cookies, cheese). You *gradually* substitute healthier foods that you like. For example, you *gradually* substitute low-fat varieties of dairy foods for the high-fat ones you may now be eating. You get plenty of advice to help you become a wise shopper and competent preparer of healthy food. And you do all this at your own pace; you decide how fast to go. We encourage you to remember that if you try to go too fast you may in the long run end up gaining rather than losing weight.

Exercise is often given short shrift in weight-loss programs. Many programs, if they talk about exercise at all, simply say, "Do it." They may give you as much instruction as "walk for 45 minutes four times a week." But you may need more than that if exercise is going to become a meaningful part of your life. Or you may not be fit enough to undertake even a 45-minute walk at the outset. You need advice on dealing with the "Oh, yuck" feelings that many people have when they think about exercising. Chapters 7, 8, and 9 will help you establish a regular exercise regimen that you can handle, one that will work for you.

Finally, this book includes several appendixes that cover background material, as well as suggested readings and general references. Because the premises and principles of the Take Control of Your Weight Program differ in certain significant ways from those of the weight-loss programs with which you are likely to be familiar, we recommend that you read chapters 1 through 3, which are devoted primarily to theory, before you read chapters 4 through 9, which are devoted primarily to practice.

However, you can safely use this program without digesting the material in the first three chapters. So, if you want to begin immediately, you can proceed directly to chapter 4, which will put you right into the program. You will pick up some of the theory from reading and implementing the practice chapters. Conversely, if you are especially interested in weight-loss theory as well as practice, in addition to the first three chapters you will want to read Appendixes A and B.

Now, let us begin this journey together.

1

Pathways to Overweight

Why You Eat

From what you hear and read these days about all the psychological factors driving one to the refrigerator, you might think that eating is a bad habit that can be cured only by extensive therapy. Of course, that is nonsense. Eating is a necessary function of life, not a compulsion. Your body uses food to repair and rebuild necessary tissue, as well as to provide you with the energy you need to go on living. In short, you eat because if you don't you will die, and the first law of nature is self-preservation. Reminding yourself of this reality may spare you the disappointment of pursuing false leads in your quest for a more attractive body.

This is not to say that you may not have developed self-destructive habits in the way you eat, or in the choice of particular foods you regularly eat. But you must understand that eating is not the enemy.

Metabolism

The *metabolic system* is the set of mechanisms the body uses to process food into biochemical fuel that provides it with the energy to support its various physical and mental functions, and to ensure safe disposal of the waste products created by the whole process. *Metabolism* is the name given to this process.

Metabolism is the key to life. But, like all processes of the body, metabolism can go awry in times of illness or stress. Because of its complexity, metabolic action sometimes produces undesirable results, even in a healthy person.

The Old Theory

Until fairly recently, conventional wisdom held that weight change followed a simple equation: Weight gain equals more calories in, fewer calories out. (A calorie is not a tangible thing, but rather a measure of the energy produced when a portion of food is metabolized.) If you ate food (calories in) that contained more calories than your body required to meet its energy needs (calories out), you gained weight; if you expended more calories than you consumed, you experienced negative gain, or loss. This being the case, the theory continued, if you were overweight and you wanted to lose, all you had to do was eat food of lower caloric value than your current energy consumption required. Your body would supply the rest of its energy needs by depleting its fat cells.

How simple! How marvelous! However, attempts to sell this theory to the general public met with divided results. Some overweight people were driven to self-loathing because of their own failures in negotiating this simple solution to their problems. Others recognized that the theory was not confirmed in their own experience, or in the experiences of many people they knew, and stopped turning to the medical and nutritional professions for advice about weight control. So was born a whole new industry devoted to innovative diet plans. It preached hope, promising a new body in so many days, while many overweight patients received from their doctors only lectures on self-discipline and a mimeographed copy of a bland-as-cardboard 1,000-calorie diet.

Unfortunately, in most cases, this new diet industry didn't do much better than the old-fashioned nutritionists. And its hope was not firmly based on complete and reliable information, leading in the end to terrible disappointment.

In recent years, nutritionists and epidemiologists have taken some giant steps in trying to solve the riddles of body weight. Although several new theories remain controversial, it is already clear that things are not nearly as simple as we once thought them to be. For example, we now know that at least some overweight people eat *less* than do many people of normal weight. This new information, which is being developed by scientific researchers, and particularly the work being done on metabolism, has been very useful in helping us understand the true causes of unwanted weight gain and successful weight loss.

Life as Motion

A first step in understanding the relationship between weight loss and eating, metabolism, and body movement is to think about life itself as nothing more, or less, than sustained motion. Consider this idea for a minute. There are the motions of muscles you consciously control—such as those of the arms and legs—and the motions of muscles under involuntary control—such as those of the heart and intestines. Thinking—what your brain is doing, for example, as you read this book—is the product of the motion of cellular and subcellular fluids and microelectrical currents. In addition to being the mechanism of voluntary and involuntary muscular action, and of thought, feelings, emotions, and creativity, some kind of motion regulates and mediates all our senses, such as vision, hearing, and touch. When motion stops, life comes to an end.

None of this motion can take place without the energy you provide your body in the food you eat. Everyone must have a certain amount of energy each day to continue this necessary motion, though we know that what constitutes a minimum or even appropriate amount of energy varies from person to person. It is important to note that it is not just the vigorous exerciser who needs energy. Daydreamers need energy to continue daydreaming. The meditator who sits quietly for hours on end needs energy to continue sitting and contemplating.

The key to understanding how life is maintained lies in understanding how food is converted into energy. And it is the metabolic system that carries out that conversion. Food, of course, has purposes other than providing energy. For example, it supplies you with the basic biochemical building blocks that the body puts together to maintain appropriate levels of its many kinds of cells, such as bone, muscle, and fluid. But even the rebuilding processes require motion, then energy, then food with sufficient caloric value to supply the energy.

Just as there is a complex interrelationship among life, motion, and energy, so are there complex interrelationships among energy, food, exercise, and the metabolic system.

Weight States as Processes

Just as life is motion, so is any given state of weight a dynamic, not static, reality. Your body is constantly renewing itself, and in doing so, changing, whether it increases, decreases, or stays the same in size. While it is true that at any given time the weights of most people are in a state of balance—whether the weight is high, low, or at a happy medium—over the years weight changes. "Normal" weight varies within individuals—for example, most of us get heavier as we get older—and it varies from one individual to another.

Recall from the introduction that overweight is not defined as weighing too much but rather as having too much extra body fat. We must now define fat.

Fat and Its Functions

Fat and Fat Cells

Fat is found in two kinds of cells—small and large fat cells. As you might imagine, they are distinguished from one another by their size. Although it was formerly thought that the number of fat cells was fixed at some time in childhood, it is now considered most likely that an increase in the number of fat cells, a condition called *hyperplastic obesity,* can occur in adulthood as well. It is also possible for the amount of fat in each fat cell to increase, enlarging the cells; this condition is called *hypertrophic obesity.*

At present, it is impossible to determine how much of any individual's weight gain is attributable to hyperplastic activity and how much to hypertrophic. However, the evidence to date is pretty clear that weight loss is the product of the loss of fat in each fat cell, not a decrease in the number of cells. It seems to be impossible to decrease the number of fat cells, once they have been created. It is well known that there are some people who can lose only a certain amount of weight, but no more, no matter how hard they try. These individuals may well have a weight gain that was primarily hyperplastic obesity. When they reduce each fat cell to its minimum size, they cannot go any further to reduce overall fat and weight. More research needs to be done to determine if it is possible to distinguish hypertrophic from hyperplastic obesity clinically.

The Functions of Body Fat

Body fat serves three primary purposes: protection from injury, protection against cold, and energy storage. Body fat shields us against mechanical injury, as do the sheaths that surround the nerves and the fat pads that protect many of our internal organs. Subcutaneous body fat (fat just beneath the skin) provides not only protection against cold, but also some mechanical protection for the musculoskeletal system and the internal organs.

Energy storage is the third function of body fat. If you consume food containing more calories than your body needs to meet its present energy requirements, your body can take that unneeded energy and store it in the form of body fat for potential future reconversion to energy. This function of body fat evolved tens of thousands of years ago when our ancestors lived by hunting and gathering. Unfortunately, while it may once have been an essential survival tool, its super efficiency has come to haunt the modern, urban human animal. Indeed, it is this too-much-of-a-good-thing aspect of this once-vital function that leads to obesity.

How the Metabolic System Creates Excess Fat

Survival and Metabolism

For our hunter-gatherer ancestors, the food supply was not always reliable. A cold winter could significantly reduce the supply of game and edible fruits and berries produced in the wild. By and large, there were no provisions for food storage in times of plenty to protect against food shortage in other times. Such periodic interruptions in the food supply threatened to make the human animal an extinct species. It is a great shame of our time that people continue to starve in many parts of the world, but today's reasons for starvation have more to do with how we handle the environment, and how the world's total food supply is distributed, than with the vagaries of nature.

In the absence of any external food storage devices, natural selection favored our ancestors who could get through periods of reduced food supply by another means: the conversion of energy-laden meals into excess body fat. The excess fat could then be turned into energy when food was in short supply. Because only those who could survive would go on to reproduce others like themselves, the ability to store energy as fat became more and more widespread among future generations.

Metabolism and Energy Storage

The body—elegantly efficient machine that it is—chooses not to waste whatever energy it has in hand. Contrast it, if you will, to the energy storage system in your car. When your car runs low on fuel, you must go to the gas station to fill up its storage tank. But that tank has a finite size. If you overfill the tank, the excess gasoline will pour out onto the ground and be wasted. Your car's gas tank cannot expand to accommodate the additional supply. But your body's energy storage system can, and does. As stated previously, the extra energy-laden fat is kept either in the subcutaneous fat layer or in the abdominal cavity, there expanding a layer of fatty tissue called the *omentum,* which protects the abdominal organs.

In metabolic terms, then, much body fat is just stored energy. Put another way, excess fat is nothing more than tomorrow's meal you ate two years ago.

Why the Storage Mechanism Favors
One Person Over Another

We know that all people, even those in the same family, don't eat the same diets. The nursery rhyme tells us of an extreme couple, Jack Sprat, who ate no fat, and his wife, who ate no lean. It doesn't take a medical school education to guess that Jack was probably thinner than Mrs. Sprat; fat carries more than twice as many calories per ounce than protein, the major component of lean meat. (The caloric ratio for protein, carbohydrate, and fat is 4:4:9.) But if you believe that this is all there is, you are in error. There is another reason that people who eat fat get fat.

When excess energy is offered to your body in the form of food fat, rather than as carbohydrate or protein, the body is very efficient at moving that excess into storage as body fat. It requires only about 3 percent of the calories in the excess food fat to move it physically into storage fat. Even if eaten in excess, both carbohydrate and protein need to be biochemically converted into fat molecules before they can be stored as body fat, a process that uses up 25 to 30 percent of the calories. Therefore, if you eat too much, it will be easier to gain weight if you are eating extra fat than if you are eating extra carbohydrate or protein, though if you eat too much of the latter two your body will be able, though less efficiently, to store the additional energy value as fat.

The Starvation Response

Two characteristics of metabolism led to increased chances of survival during periods of food shortage. We have just spoken of one—the ability to store extra energy on the body itself when food was abundant. The other is the body's ability to reduce its resting metabolic rate when food is in short supply. This process is called the *starvation response*. Unfortunately, like the first, this marvelous device designed by nature to aid survival in harder times contributes to obesity in our food-rich society.

The starvation response kicks in when you suddenly reduce your caloric intake, as you do in most sudden-weight-loss diets. Using another mechanism developed in our hunter-gatherer days, your body reads the failure to take in new food as a threat to its ultimate survival. It concludes "Oh my gosh, the hunt failed," or perhaps "Did the birds eat *all* the berries this year?" Being very clever about these things, the body decides that it must take quick steps (*very* quick steps, it turns out) to conserve energy.

It begins this process by reducing its resting metabolic rate. This is the rate at which your body consumes energy to keep the basic systems—cardiac, respiratory, digestive, and so forth—functioning. The RMR has a built-in flexibility, no doubt itself the product of evolutionary selection. Your body can easily reduce its RMR by half and still survive quite well. An extreme example of this process in the animal kingdom is hibernation, in which certain animals severely depress their metabolic systems and go into deep sleep through food-scarce winters. In humans, the slow-down process appears to begin within 36 to 48 hours after any sudden reduction in caloric intake.

Calorie-Restriction Dieting and the Starvation Response

The modern American trigger for the starvation response is not the failure of a hunt or an important crop, but the start of an aggressive calorie-restriction diet. Let's follow the confusing signals the human body was given by a hypothetical dieter named Kim.

Having decided to lose some weight, Kim went on a 14-day low-calorie wonder diet. Although she was not eating too much before starting the diet, she managed to lose some weight by rigorously following the diet's prescriptions and dramatically cutting down on her caloric intake. Her body attempted to conserve its energy by reducing its RMR, but Kim, watching her scale daily, kept reducing caloric intake until she reached her desired weight-loss goal. Ah, success! How good it feels!

Having received nothing more than the most general advice on how to eat in a healthy manner after she reached her diet goals, Kim gradually returned to her old eating habits. She thought she'd be all right. She didn't want to lose any more weight, and this level of eating would keep her weight fairly stable.

But Kim's daily visits to her scale gradually became occasions for panic. Eating no more than she did before she began her diet, she watched in horror as her weight climbed and climbed, wiping out all her dearly purchased progress. Although she ate no more than what once kept her stabilized at a higher weight, her weight soon exceeded what it was before her diet.

Why did this happen? Before she started the diet, Kim's weight, although elevated, had been stable for quite some time, as had been her eating pattern. Kim's weight, though higher than she preferred it to be, was stable because her energy demands and caloric intake were both stable, and the body had had a chance to adjust the RMR to maintain the balance. (The body's attempt to stabilize weight by adjusting the RMR based on caloric intake is sometimes called the *set-point theory*. We shall consider it in some detail later in this chapter.)

As Kim started the diet, her body didn't judge itself as overweight. It didn't know that it was already carrying plenty of extra energy stored as body fat and that on the diet Kim planned it could have made up for any energy shortfall solely by drawing on stored fat. Thus, when Kim's body read "sudden restriction in available calories," it responded by triggering the starvation response. While drawing on stored fat for the short term, it started adjusting its RMR downward until it could maintain a constant weight without using any more of its stored reserves.

Now, you might ask, when Kim went back to her regular diet, why didn't the body read that as an indication that the food emergency was over and reset the RMR? Because, unfortunately, the body is not equipped to read the second signal. Remember, the starvation response was developed through natural selection as an adaptation to long-term, not short-term, food shortages. And survival of the species required that the body err on the safe side. Once the body's fat stores were exhausted, and there was still no food available, it would be too late to go back and do a better job of conserving energy.

After Kim finished the diet and went back to her regular eating habits, her body continued to play it cautiously. It kept the RMR down and began to replace the stored reserves it had lost during the emergency. Once bitten, twice shy, goes an old saying, and Kim's body continued to be pessimistic about the future availability of food, even when her levels of stored fat were greater than they had been at the beginning of the perceived emergency. Acting contrary to Kim's wishes, her body continued to respond to the food-scarcity cues it had received when the diet began, rebuilding its fat stores from the excess calories it was now taking in as part of the regular, pre-diet, eating pattern. This was possible because at the body's newly lowered resting metabolic rate, some of those calories that had been previously used to meet energy needs were now available for storage.

With every good intention, Kim used a weight-loss program that simply could not, for metabolic reasons, help to meet a long-term goal of losing weight and keeping it off. Although Kim might have been consumed with guilt at the chaotic end of her weight-loss plan, the fault was not Kim's. That lies with the failure of the designer of the diet plan to take account of how the human body responds to such assaults on its equilibrium.

Is Fat Sinful?

In our culture excess body fat has been characterized as immoral, both by some overweight people themselves and by certain others (see Appendix B). This characterization is harmful, both to the overweight person and to the weight-loss process itself. Body fat is many things, but an understanding of its metabolism and evolutionary origins shows us that having an excess of it is hardly immoral or sinful. Being overweight does not mean that you have fallen from a state of grace. How useful it would be if we could rid the language of those phrases that link being overweight and eating excess fat to morality:

"Doesn't that chocolate cake look *sinful*?"

"I was *bad*. I had a hot-fudge sundae last night."
"I wish I could be *good,* and stay away from fattening food."

Or those that pose fat as an enemy:

"I'm getting *so* tired of *fighting* my fat."

Fat is not a sin or sinful, neither is it your enemy. As we have seen, it has helped the human species survive its early difficult history. Like most good things in life, of course, you can get too much of it. But fat is not mystical. It's not magical. It is just, well, fat.

Set-Point Theory

In discussions on metabolism, fat, and obesity, since the early 1980s there has been a lot of attention given to something called the set-point theory. Among its original developers were William Bennett, M.D., and Joel Gurin *(The Dieter's Dilemma)* and Dennis Remington *(How to Lower Your Fat Thermostat)*. From their reviews of the literature, they concluded that each person's body has a sort of thermostat that controls his or her weight. After each weight loss this thermostat will induce the body to return to its original weight, regardless of what changes the person imposes on his or her body. A weight-control center in the brain is thought to "choose" the amount of body fat necessary to meet the body's needs and then it works to maintain that level. The chosen weight/fat level is called the *set point.*

Set-Point Controversy

There seems little doubt that for each of us, *at any one time,* there is a weight, or set point, to which we will return after weight loss. Everyone who has lost weight on one diet or another and who has returned to his or her previous weight or gained more weight, will attest to this. But is each person's set point fixed, or is it variable over time? And if it is variable, can we consciously change or control it?

According to William Bennett, it is "fixed, not variable. No intervention has been shown consistently to achieve true weight control, as opposed to temporary weight loss. . . . Circumstantial evidence now clearly suggests that in the long run both food intake and body fat are consequences of the equilibrium in a complex system . . . obesity cannot be reliably prevented or reversed. . . ."

However, Martin Katahn, Ph.D., director of the Vanderbilt (University) Weight Management Program and author of *The T-Factor Diet,* disagrees vigorously with William Bennett's opinion and believes that the set point is "variable, and yes, changeable by intervention." He believes the fixed set-point theory is a "most unfortunate misconception," both because it discourages people from attempting to lose weight and because it is incorrect. He has concluded from his studies that there is not just *one* set point for each of us, but many, representing *"a range of adaptability."* Inside the limits of that range, alterations in diet and exercise can easily and conveniently be effective in achieving permanent weight loss.

The weight of evidence seems to be on Dr. Katahn's side. As stated above, the body does behave at times as if it had something like a set point, though that point also appears to be quite variable over time. Consider the experience of Everyperson, for example, who was at normal weight (had a stable set point) until his or her late twenties, and then either became pregnant with a first child or took on a high-stress job or underwent some life change that encouraged overeating. Everyperson then gained weight until he or she stabilized at a new weight level. When Everyperson's later attempts to lose this weight ran into stubborn resistance, someone offered the set-point theory as explanation. No matter what Everyperson did, the explanation went, the moment he or she relaxed, the body would return to a certain weight, its set point.

Can the Set Point Be Lowered?

It stands to reason that if Everyperson's original set point (which had determined a normal weight) was modified upward, as it must have been as he or she settled so comfortably into all that extra weight, then it should be possible to lower the set point to produce weight loss.

It is helpful to understand how the set point is modified upward in the first place. In overweight that results from stimulation of the starvation response by calorie-restrictive dieting, the set point goes up because the resting metabolic rate goes down. It stands to reason that to lower the set point, the body's RMR would have to be raised back up toward normal. That is not easy, but it can be done. Most authorities now agree that the only known way of doing it is to undertake regular exercise.

Some people are very comfortable with the notion that each person's set point is fixed, immutable. It fits in well with the thinking of those who urge overweight people to accept their bodies as they are. Most overweight is genetically determined, goes the argument, and since 95 percent of dieters fail anyway, trying isn't worth the bother. The overweight can forget about losing weight and get to work on becoming happy with themselves as they are. The set-point theory helps them rationalize such a decision.

The Take Control of Your Weight Program finds itself in tune with at least some aspects of the statement "Diets don't work." Acute calorie-restriction diets, by themselves, definitely don't work. Also, through the starvation response such diets can easily lead to regaining the lost weight, leading then to a succession of diets and the yo-yo pattern of weight loss and gain, and eventually to long-term weight gain. However, as the experiences of many people have shown, weight-loss approaches that combine healthy eating with regular exercise, in a pattern of gradual change custom-designed for the person who wants to lose weight and keep it off, *do* work. We believe that your chances for success are improved when *you* are your own plan's custom designer.

The Pathways Up to Overweight

It should now be clear that we do not reach obesity by just one route. It is not as simple as calories in, calories out. Current understanding of metabolism tells us that there are several different pathways that people take to go from normal weight to overweight.

To repeat, overweight is produced by an imbalance among the amount and type of food you eat, the amount of energy you expend, *and* the activity level of your metabolic system. The following are the four major Pathways Up to overweight (other than disease-induced overweight, which we do not cover in this book):

- Overeating
- Familial induction
- Genetic predisposition
- Weight-loss-diet induction

Each pathway represents a different cause and type of overweight. On each pathway people have different metabolic functioning, different food intakes, different food requirements.

The knowledge of your metabolism that you have acquired by reading this chapter should enable you to understand each of the four pathways better. Unfortunately, no epidemiological studies have been done to determine the distribution of obesity in the population among these four types of weight gain. It is unimportant to your own progress to know the exact statistics. What is important is identifying which type you are.

The Types of Overweight

Overeating is what it sounds like. The person is simply eating too much in terms of his or her energy requirements. This may be a short- or a long-term phenomenon. The person's weight will continue to rise until either the overeating is consciously brought under control, or a state of equilibrium is reached at a high weight.

Family-induced (or familial) *overweight* usually begins in childhood. Family life during childhood may have often centered around eating. The food placed on the table was high in calories and served in ample quantities. Often, the parents were overweight. In many cases, food was given as a reward for good behavior. Eating was a way for the child to show approval or appreciation to both food provider and preparer.

The person with familial overweight has remained heavy, and may have engaged in few, if any, attempts to lose weight. Presently he or she is often in caloric balance, eating in the normal range, with the body adjusting RMR to maintain an elevated but stable weight.

Genetically predisposed and *diet-induced overweight* are related in that both can occur in the absence of high-calorie eating. The general term for these two types of overweight is *low-calorie overweight* (LCO).

In genetically predisposed LCO, there is some genetic, inherited factor that depresses the resting metabolic rate (RMR), or otherwise alters metabolism and leads to overweight. If the mechanism is indeed a lowered RMR, the scenario is similar to that which follows the stimulation of the starvation response, but is built in to the person's metabolism from birth, even though it may not be triggered until adulthood.

The diet-induced LCO is created not by an inherited predisposition to a lower RMR but the triggering of the starvation response following sudden calorie-restrictive dieting. Although we don't know for sure, given the involvement of this country's population with weight-loss attempts, and the popularity of sudden calorie-restriction diets promising immediate gratification in terms of pounds lost, diet-induced LCO may be the most common type of overweight in the United States.

Later in this book you will learn how to determine which Pathway Up you took to overweight, so that you can select the Pathway Down that provides you with the best prospects for success. But before you get into designing your program, you will have to understand the most important first step in any weight-loss program: goal setting.

2

Motivation and Goals

What Is Motivation?

Motivation, a concept central to weight loss, is often imprecisely understood. We frequently say, or hear others say, "I've got to get motivated," or "My motivation is high right now," but sometimes we have difficulty putting into words the exact meaning of the term when we use or hear it. You should find the following working definition helpful when reading this chapter.

Motivation is a state of mind characterized as an emotion, feeling, desire, idea, or intellectual understanding, or a psychological, physiological, or health need mediated by a conscious or unconscious mental process that leads to the taking of one or more actions.

Note that the root of the word "motivation," *motive,* has two meanings. Originally, it meant *moving.* It later developed its additional modern meaning, *the dominant factor in the mental process that causes a person to act.* The relevant points are that motivation is always related to movement, or action, and that it is not something that can be given to you, or caught from another, but must always take place within your own mind.

Motivation is mobilizing; lack of it is immobilizing, often paralyzing. When we talk about either "being motivated" or "lacking motivation" to lose weight, we are referring to various states of mind that will, or will not, impel us to undertake action that we believe will take us to our goal. Further, when we talk about "finding" or "developing" motivation, we are talking about (1) experiencing certain emotional and intellectual processes; (2) establishing a clear pathway between those processes and the related action; and (3) taking action as the result of being pushed to do so by these mental processes.

The ultimate question the potential weight-loser must answer is, "Am I going to change, or am I not going to change—really?" Positive change cannot occur in the absence of an emotional and/or intellectual commitment to bring about change, that is, motivation.

Is Positive Change Possible?

Motivation has many elements. Initially, mobilizing for successful weight loss requires that you believe that successful weight loss is possible for you. We discussed this belief earlier, as it applied to whether or not the chances of long-term success are good enough to justify the investment in time and effort that a weight-loss program requires. Here, we will deal with that belief again, but from a different perspective. Even if all the medical studies ever done in this field strongly supported the position that long-term weight loss is indeed possible for most people—and not all studies strongly support this position—your chances for success would still be low if you were not convinced that success is possible for *you*.

As we noted previously, many studies describe the low success rates of participants in organized weight-loss programs. These numbers understandably discourage many people who would like to lose weight, and lead them to question very seriously whether or not they should make the attempt. It is not entirely unreasonable to think, If I have as little as a one-in-twenty shot at making it, why should I even bother?

But, remember that the commonly quoted low success rates represent people who enter supervised weight-loss programs. Admittedly, the data on the rate of success in self-directed weight loss is very skimpy. One study, by Stanley Schachter, examined people who had tried to lose weight on their own, and found a success rate of about 60 percent. More research needs to be done. But what we have points in a positive direction. Losing weight successfully is possible for significant numbers of people. Many, especially among those who make the attempt on their own, have been successful.

Still, all the studies in the world will have no effect on your chances for success unless you believe that you will be among the 60 percent or so who do achieve success on their own.

Weight Loss and Addictive Behavior:
Implications for Success

In the view of most, although not all, weight-loss authorities, overweight is *not* the result of addictive behavior, at least not in most overweight people. It is not helpful, and may be cruel, to tell people who are unhappy with their weight that they are food addicts. However, it may be possible to learn something from professionals who treat people trying to change addictive behavior such as *inappropriate* drug use or compulsive gambling. The evidence is clear that earlier pessimism regarding the prognosis for the typical addict was not warranted; many addicted people do eventually come to control their addictive behavior if their personal motivation to do so is strong enough. More to the point of this book, most people who end or change their addictive behavior do so on their own. Sound familiar?

To lose weight and keep it off, you may need to make major alterations in life-style similar to the changes that people addicted to other destructive behavior must make (even though overweight is usually not the result of addictive behavior). The overweight person, especially the overeater, must change eating patterns, and most overweight people, regardless of how they got there, must engage in regular exercise of some type before they can hope to bring about positive and permanent changes in body weight.

Motivation and the Process of Change

A useful model of the process through which motivation brings about positive change was developed by the psychologists James Prochaska and Carlo DiClemente. The two identified eight stages of the motivation process (subsequently refined to fewer). Here we shall consider five of the eight stages: precontemplation, contemplation, determination, action, and maintenance.

Precontemplation

You have not yet determined that you have a problem that requires remedy. If you are overweight, you are aware of the fact but accept the state of affairs, happily or unhappily.

Contemplation

This is the stage in which you recognize that you have a problem or a condition about which you want to do something. But the prospect that you might make a change has not yet progressed beyond a generalized "I'm thinking about it."

At least part of your mind is in favor of making changes and of doing something serious about achieving them. But often, another part of your mind is not completely convinced. This conflict is called ambivalence.

Ambivalence. Ambivalence is the state of mind in which contradictory feelings about your contemplated action coexist. This stage is perfectly normal before a commitment to any change. Virtually everyone who ever thinks about making any major alteration in the way his or her life is organized experiences conflicted feelings. Handling them the right way can help you get started down the path to weight loss.

You must accept that reasons for not embarking on a program will always be floating around in your mind, screaming for a hearing, as will those feelings later on that will be telling you that you've gone far enough and it's time to quit. At times these ambivalent feelings will be weaker, at other times stronger. Don't fight them. In fact, the more fully and openly you deal with them at this early stage, the less they will trouble you later. The more you suppress them now, the more you will be inclined at some future date to grind your program to a halt and go back and question whether or not you ever gave sufficient consideration to those negative whisperings.

Before starting, you have to get as many parts of your brain on board as possible, though some grumbling by the ambivalent crew may continue. You do not have to resolve your ambivalence completely in order to leave the station, but there must be a strong consensus within you that states forcefully and credibly, "Yes, I would like to change; yes, I *can* change."

Once you have started on a program, and you encounter the feelings again, you will be able to remind yourself that you have gone over this ground, that you have given a fair hearing to the cons as well as the pros, and that your original decision to proceed is as valid now as it was then. This will help prevent your stalling the program and undoing what you have accomplished.

Determination

In the Prochaska/DiClemente model, the next stage in the motivation/change process is called determination. When you have entered this stage, you have, in common parlance, "become motivated." You possess those thoughts, emotions, and rational considerations that overcome your ambivalent feelings and doubts and persuade you that you can succeed. There are several ways to achieve determination; some work well, some don't.

Self-confrontation. Among the ways that don't work well are those that can be classified as self-confrontational. Self-confrontation usually involves attitudes such as *have to, ought to,* or *should,* in contrast with *want to* and *would like to.* Declarations that you have to, ought to, or should do something depend on guilt for their success. We know from past experience that we can expect feelings of self-reproach to overwhelm us when we fail to do something that we have to, ought to, or should do. Therefore, it seems logical that you would go ahead and do what you should in order to avoid the unpleasant feelings associated with guilt.

However, guilt feelings, whether coming from ourselves or induced by others, don't work very well as motivators. Guilt elicits resistance or denial, translated as "I don't wanna," and "Problem? What problem?"

Furthermore, guilt about anything we have done or intend to do leads not to reform but to frustration and anger. Because we don't like feeling either angry or frustrated, we are likely to reject any action that leads to those feelings. We abandon our intent to lose weight because it necessitates that we focus on a plan and the reasons behind it. No matter how well it seems to work in the beginning, guilt—the "you-gotta" approach—is counterproductive in the end. Don't do it to yourself, and don't let others do it to you.

Pleasing others. Externally generated motivation does not work for most people. If you decide to try to lose weight to please others—spouse, parents, children, boss, employees, co-workers, or even the general public—you will not succeed. Wanting to have a better physical image only because you wish to impress other people will not sufficiently motivate you to lose weight permanently. As with guilt feelings, this attitude often leads to resentment, frustration, anger, and failure. You start off thinking, I'm going to do it for so-and-so and so-and-so, because they love me and it would please them. Later, you get to, That's a lot they expect me to do for them, just so they won't be ashamed of me. Finally it's, If they don't like me the way I am, tough!

Losing weight and keeping it off will take you down an often lonely and always highly personal road. To succeed, you must want to make the trip primarily for yourself. Research into motivation has shown that intrinsic, or self-generated, motivation works best.

Self-motivation. Whereas guilt and pleasing others are counterproductive, the desire to feel good about yourself, for yourself, is most productive. A goal of self-satisfaction—not the desire to avoid censure—is the key to successful motivation. In turn, self-motivation is the key to inner determination.

If you want to look better, feel healthier, be fitter, and feel better about yourself, for yourself and no one else, then you already have inner determination. If you view the praise of others as no more than a fringe benefit, you have inner determination. You are ready to start taking control of the way you eat and exercise. The chances are excellent that you will be able to lose weight, gradually and carefully, and keep it off.

Action

The next step in the process of change is the commitment to action. Without this commitment, all motivating thoughts are sterile. The process by which you convert determination into action isn't always clear. One moment you may be building your resolve to get started, and the next you are looking around for the first step to take, sometimes too impatient for the sun to rise so that you can begin. You'll know when you are ready to begin. If you aren't sure when you want to start, or even *if* you want to start, you have not yet reached the point of action. If you are thinking, Let's get on with it, let's hear how the Take Control of Your Weight Program works so I can get started on my own program, you are ready to begin.

Maintenance

Maintenance is the final step in the process of change and the one you want to reach. Once you enter the program you want to continue to be motivated to stay with it to a successful end. Once you have lost weight, you want to keep it off, permanently. There are three possible departures from the maintenance stage: lapse, relapse, and permanent exit.

Lapse. Lapse is a *temporary* abandonment of the positive behavior that has helped you to lose weight: having a hot fudge sundae, eating a thick steak made juicy and tender by all the marbleized fat that runs through it, or taking a couple of weeks off from your regular exercise program. Lapse, because it is temporary, seldom produces any significant alteration in your progress toward your goals or any significant backslide after you have achieved them. The key words are *temporary* and *significant*.

For example, you have lost 10 pounds over a month or two toward a goal of a 30-pound weight loss in six months. Regaining a pound or two after eating a high-fat meal is not significant. It happens to most weight-losers. Once you've lost the 30 pounds, you need not worry if you lapse into your previous eating pattern and regain 5 of those pounds, stop there, and return to your new healthy eating pattern. Your taste and tolerance for fatty foods, which are always the cause of dietary lapse, will diminish over time as you eat less and less of them. Taking an occasional rest from regular exercise is actually advisable for most of us.

Lapse is fine, lapse can be fun and is perfectly normal. However, if the lapse ceases to be temporary, much more significant damage will be done.

Relapse. You are in relapse if you abandon your positive behavior patterns to the extent that you regain a significant portion or all of your weight loss. The good feelings you experienced while losing that weight disappear. The first step in reversing relapse is to figure out why the relapse occurred. Then you must go back to the contemplation stage and start the motivation-for-change process all over again.

It is important to understand that neither overweight nor relapse is a sign of moral failure or weakness. Relapse simply means that you weren't really ready the first time around, that you were not really motivated in a way that would work for you, and perhaps that your goals were unrealistic.

Even before you start the weight-loss process, you should be aware of some predictors of relapse. For example, "I need someone to tell me what to do. I need specifics in menus, meal plans, what foods to eat, etc." Just as external motivation doesn't work in the long run, neither does external direction. Maintenance of a lower weight requires a permanent change in your eating and exercise patterns. Very few people will follow a diet book for the rest of their lives. No one continues to eat according to external direction; only healthy eating and activity that is built into your regular living patterns will keep the weight off. To maintain your new weight, you will have to internalize healthy patterns of shopping, cooking, eating, and exercise and make them routine, as routine as the patterns of eating and activity that led to your overweight in the first place.

Another tell-tale sign of future failure could be "I need to lose a lot of weight quickly for (you name it) the wedding, the bar mitzvah, the bikini season." If you have not done so before, you may be able to achieve your short-term goal by sudden calorie restriction. But even if you are successful, that process always leads to the starvation response. And, as you know by now, the starvation response always leads to weight regain.

And then there is "I need a new diet—that's the answer." You may very well need a new *approach* to weight loss. But, as we know, specific diets don't work over time, not only because many of them unbalance your metabolic processes, but also because external direction doesn't work for very long.

If you go into relapse, it is important that you don't let your natural disappointment turn to discouragement or demoralization. Remember that there are often good reasons for relapse. It happens to many people—good people, strong people—and doesn't mean that you won't eventually achieve your goals. Once you do, you'll experience permanent exit.

Permanent exit. Permanent exit means that you have sufficiently changed your eating and exercise patterns so that you adhere to the new ways without much conscious thought or effort. You may have lapsed along the way. Who hasn't? In fact, lapsing can be fun (if you don't overdo it and end up feeling awful from eating too much fat, or with significant muscle pain when you go back to regular exercise after a too-long layoff). You don't have to be perfect to stay in control and keep your body in the shape that you like. Occasional lapsing can contribute to maintaining permanent exit by avoiding rigidity and perfectionism, which, in the long run, can be more damaging.

But you do not relapse, you do not lose any significant portion of your physical or psychological gains, and you continue going forward. Once you have reached your goals, permanent exit defines successful weight loss.

Strategies for Strengthening Motivation

Among those who successfully make the journey all the way to permanent exit, the most common reply to the question, "How did you get started?" is "I just decided to do it." But there are a number of factors that can make your decision work for you.

Establishing Your Knowledge Base

Establishing a knowledge base is also called "achieving cognitive understanding." You have learned how and why people gain weight, how they can lose weight, and how metabolism can make losing weight extremely difficult or impossible. You have learned the risks and benefits of remaining overweight, and the benefits and risks of losing weight. You carry out your own risk/benefit analysis, learning and understanding why change is important. You will be increasing your appreciation of why a decision *not* to make a change is *not* desirable for you. An important part of your knowledge base is the understanding that the process of change is not simple. It takes a lot of thought, organization, and determination.

Providing Yourself with Choices

The most central strategy for motivation is to provide yourself with choices. And you have many choices, including whether to undertake a change process at all, what goal you are going to set for yourself, which method to use. *Take Control of Your Weight* stresses a method that requires you to make many choices and puts *you* in charge. Making choices, of course, means taking responsibility for yourself. Taking control, taking responsibility, and having plenty of choices are powerful motivational tools.

Dealing with the Need for Immediate Gratification

Immediate gratification or the promise of it is a common element of contemporary American society. You are continually urged to let yourself go and indulge in immedite gratification in many ways. For example, you are told that if you suddenly crave a certain burger, you must immediately go out and satisfy that hunger, regardless of what else is going on in your life at the time. Immediate gratification is also offered by the instant scratch-off games in various public and private lotteries. No need to wait. You will know right away if you are a winner.

And isn't our consumer-oriented economy built on immediate gratification? You want the new car, new TV, new camcorder, or other big-ticket item right now, don't you? Don't have the money? Not to worry. Don't even think about waiting until you have saved up for it. Just put it on the card. The federal government borrows all the time, in larger and larger amounts; so do major corporations. You can do it too, and you can get what you want right away, before you change your mind about wanting it.

You are also promised immediate gratification by any of the three-week wonder diets. In a society that promotes immediate gratification, and in a weight-loss environment that focuses on scale weight, how can you make wise choices about weight loss? Well, you may use cognitive reasoning if you understand where the desire for instant gratification comes from and that it can only harm you, not help you.

Rather, let immediate gratification come from your mind, not from scale weight. For example, there is immediate gratification in taking control, taking responsibility, empowering yourself, and doing something new and different for yourself. The Take Control program offers this kind of immediate gratification.

After only a week or two on the Take Control of Your Weight Program, without any significant physical changes yet apparent, you may think, Wow, I can really do this. I can learn something about nutrition and metabolism. I can figure out what kind of overweight I have. I can design a program that suits me. And I can get on this program and look forward to staying on it. These kinds of thoughts may occur even during the preprogram planning phase. That's immediate gratification of the most positive kind.

Dealing with Perfectionism

Perfectionism is the bane of the weight-loss process. *Perfect* is defined as "complete in all respects; without defect or omission; sound; flawless." The striving for bodily perfection is socially induced (see Appendix B); it is not the product of a natural biological drive. Neither a perfect body nor a perfect mind is essential for individual or species survival.

Objectively, it should be clear that it is virtually impossible for most people to achieve a perfect body, however perfection is defined. Overweight people who make such an achievement their goal doom themselves to certain discouragement, despair, and inevitable relapse. The ultimate result for many will be either the development of an eating disorder, such as bulimia or anorexia (see Appendix B), or total disintegration of the weight-loss program as frustration and anger make further progress impossible.

As well as being the bane of weight loss, perfectionism is the enemy of the movement that promotes self-acceptance for the overweight. The promotion of an ideal body shape makes self-acceptance for the overweight person difficult. Consistent with its commitment to personal choice, the Take Control program concedes the right of the overweight person to be overweight, if that choice is freely and rationally made. Ironically, recognition that overweight is okay and is not something to feel guilty or ashamed about may be a first necessary step to successful weight loss, especially for people who had trouble losing weight in the past.

Sound principles of motivation require that you work toward a final body shape that can be realized in a reasonable amount of time with a reasonable amount of effort. Two truisms of all attempts at weight loss or management are that no one can ever achieve the perfect body, and that virtually everyone can achieve a better body.

Goals and Objectives

After you have gained an understanding of the weight-gain/weight-loss process, and after you have mobilized yourself, you must establish clear, realistic, and attainable goals before you get into the details of program planning and implementation. You must be clear about what you want to do, and why you want to do it.

A *goal* is a general statement of something that you desire to achieve. For example, "I would like to look better, feel healthier, and feel better about myself."

An *objective* is a specific measurable outcome that you can achieve within a stated time period. For example, "Within six months, I will have lost 20 pounds and 2 inches off my waist."

The Importance of Setting Goals and Objectives

"What I want to do is lose weight. What's all this about goals and objectives? Why don't we just get on with it?"

These are logical questions that many people ask. But before you can design a sound plan to get you from here to anywhere else it is essential that you clearly identify where you want to be. You may find that many people who failed to complete weight-loss programs did not set goals. It is highly likely that most people who successfully lost weight had a pretty good idea of their goal.

Think about it. When you were in high school or college, didn't your academic performance improve significantly if you had specific reasons for taking a course and knew what you wanted to get out of the experience? When there is a task to do, don't you usually do it better if you know what the goals and objectives are? Perhaps your performance even improved if you were involved in establishing the goals and objectives. Think about doing your Saturday morning chores. Don't things go better when you have a plan, when you know what you need to accomplish and how much time you have to do it in?

Goal Setting and Realism

Realism is one of the most important elements in establishing a goal. Not many of us can look like Cher or Arnold Schwarzenegger. Strong genetic components influence body shape and size in the same ways that they determine facial features. Genetics also determine whether or not you can significantly increase the bulk of your muscles. You must set personal *attainable* goals.

Of course, not everyone who is overweight wants to be fashionably thin. Nor can everyone physically and metabolically get back to what they consider their "normal" weight—what they used to weigh in college, for example. Some weight-losers will be able to attain the normal weight range for their height, body build, and age. For others, just being "less fat" will do very nicely. They will be quite content to lose some pounds and keep them off, without worrying about whether or not their new weight qualifies as normal by some medical charts.

Intermediate Goals and Objectives

How fast you lose weight is important, but from a new perspective. You should plan to lose weight slowly, not quickly, and over long stretches of time. Slow but steady is best; gradual change leads to permanent change.

Keeping this in mind, you may decide first to set intermediate goals and objectives for weight, size, eating, and exercise. It makes good sense to do this—you can decide later whether or not you want to go further. Let's take Charlie as an example.

At 6 feet 2 inches, Charlie weighed 347 pounds. He had been heavy since his teenage years. There had always been plenty of food at home. His mother was a fine cook who took great pride in her culinary skills, which featured heaping plates of fatty foods, breads spread with pure creamery butter, and salads dripping in oil and vinegar. The best way to keep on his mother's good side was to praise her food and eat plenty of it. Charlie's loving, rather round wife followed a similar style of food preparation.

Nevertheless, at age 37, Charlie decided that the time had come to lose some weight. His father, also a large man, had just had his first heart attack at age 60. Charlie's older brother, although 20 pounds lighter than Charlie, had been having increasing "trouble getting around" for the last three years. According to the tables, "normal" weight for Charlie would be about 200 pounds. That would mean losing over 40 percent of his total weight—a daunting task, to say the least.

Charlie decided to go for half the loaf. He set an intermediate goal for himself of 275 pounds. He also decided that if he could get there, and stay there, it would be fine if he also decided that it was just too much work to go the rest of the way. After all, he told himself, half a loaf is better than none. If, after getting to 275, he found that going further met his needs and desires and was within his comfort zone and capabilities, he would commit himself to a new goal at that time.

Measures of Success

In setting your goals and objectives, several variables can be considered measures of success:

- *Pounds*. Yes. But remember that only weight loss that consists primarily of fat is healthy. To lose muscle mass (the only other source of weight readily available to be lost) is unhealthy. That's another reason that calorie restriction alone is a poor way to lose weight; it causes indiscriminate loss of both fat and muscle mass.
- *Inches*. Inch loss can be a sensible objective. You can lose inches almost anywhere. If you are exercising at a moderately vigorous level, you will be building muscle and may lose inches before you lose much weight. Visible progress will help support your continued commitment.
- *Proportion of body fat*. Low-fat eating and exercise can lead to a significant decrease in your body fat without much weight loss at all, because

you are building muscle. Your proportion of body fat will be difficult for you to determine on your own, but it can be measured accurately by several kinds of health-care professionals, including your doctor.

• *Physical conditioning.* You may decide that your goal is to become physically fit, in terms of strength, endurance, and flexibility, and that your weight is a problem to you only because it interferes with achieving the fitness goal. Your measure of success will then be in terms of fitness, not in pounds. Losing weight will probably be a pleasant, but secondary, consequence.

• *Clothing fit.* This is a good measure of success without having to count pounds or inches. You will know you are making progress when you go into the back of your closet and retrieve some favorite clothes you haven't been able to wear for years.

• *Feeling good about yourself.* An increase in self-esteem resulting from whatever progress you make, in whatever area, may be your most valuable reward.

How Heavy Is Too Heavy?

According to the Take Control philosophy, there is no one level of overweight (except of morbid obesity) that is too heavy for everyone. There is no one level of normal weight that's right for everyone. What is too heavy at one stage of life may be fine at another. While one weight-loss goal may be appropriate for one stage of life, a person might try to achieve a different goal later on. Intermediate goals are fine for some people.

We believe that the following criteria—objective, subjective, and social—and discussion can help you to decide how heavy is too heavy for you.

Objective Criteria

Several different objective answers may be given to the question of how heavy is too heavy. You may find one or more of the following to be helpful:

• Too heavy might mean weighing 20 percent or more above the upper limit of your normal weight shown in Table I.1 on page 9. Your risk for various diseases and conditions, such as hypertension and diabetes, increases at 20 percent overweight. You can be too heavy if you are 50 pounds or more overweight, regardless of your height and age.

• Too heavy might mean having a body mass index (BMI) in excess of 30. The BMI is a measure of weight/height relationship, and can give you a good

TABLE 2.1 *Body Weights in Pounds According to Height and Body Mass Index*†*

Height, in Inches	Body Mass Index, kg/m²					
	19	**20**	**21**	**22**	**23**	**24**
	Body Weight, in Pounds					
58	90	95	100	105	109	114
59	93	96	103	108	113	118
60	97	102	107	112	117	122
61	100	105	110	116	121	126
62	103	109	114	120	125	130
63	107	112	118	123	129	135
64	110	116	122	127	133	139
65	113	119	125	131	137	143
66	117	123	129	136	142	148
67	121	127	133	140	146	152
68	124	131	137	144	151	157
69	128	135	141	148	155	162
70	132	139	146	153	160	166
71	135	143	150	157	164	171
72	139	147	154	161	169	176
73	143	151	158	166	174	181
74	147	155	163	171	173	186
75	151	159	167	175	183	191
76	155	164	172	180	188	196

*Each entry gives the body weight in pounds for a person of a given height and body mass index.

†Desirable body mass index range in relation to age (from Bray[2]).

Source: National Institutes of Health, Technology Assessment Conference Statement, *Methods for Voluntary Loss and Control,* March 30–April 1, 1992

idea of your body-fat proportion. You can calculate your BMI using Table 2.1. For example, a person who is 5 feet 6 inches and weighs 136 pounds has a BMI of 22, according to the table. The normal range is 19 to 27.

		Body Mass Index, kg/m²					
25	26	27	28	29	30	35	40

		Body Weight, in Pounds					
119	124	128	133	138	143	167	191
123	128	133	138	143	148	172	197
127	132	136	143	148	153	178	204
132	137	142	147	153	158	184	211
136	141	147	152	158	163	191	218
140	146	152	157	163	169	197	225
145	151	157	162	168	174	203	232
149	155	161	167	173	179	209	239
154	160	166	173	179	185	216	247
159	165	172	178	184	191	223	254
164	170	177	183	190	196	229	262
168	175	182	189	196	202	236	270
173	180	187	194	201	206	243	278
178	186	193	200	207	214	250	286
183	191	198	206	213	220	257	294
189	196	204	211	219	226	264	302
194	202	209	217	225	233	272	310
199	207	215	223	231	239	279	319
205	213	221	229	237	245	286	327

• Too heavy might be a waist-to-hip ratio (WHR) above 1. WHR is the ratio of your waist measurement (in inches) to your hip measurement (in inches). It gives you a good approximation of your proportion of abdominal fat. Among overweight people, high abdominal fat proportion (the apple shape) is more likely to lead to health risks associated with obesity than is a concentration of excess weight around the hips and on the thighs (the pear shape). An apple shape would be characterized, for example, by a waist measurement of 46 inches and a hip measurement of 42 inches (and a resulting WHR of 1.1). Apple shape is more common in men and pear shape is more common in women. If you have an apple shape and decide to lose weight, you will be happy to know that abdominal fat is usually the first to go.

● Too heavy is being a little overweight if you have a preexisting condition or disease for which obesity is a risk factor, such as adult-onset diabetes, hypertension, or osteoarthritis in the lower extremities.

Subjective Criteria

In addition to the objective measures for too heavy, there are important subjective measures such as the following:

● How do you feel? Yes, as simple as that. Do you feel fat, uncomfortable, unhappy about your weight, your size, your shape? If the answer is yes, it is a good idea to determine, perhaps by asking a friend or family member, if your feelings are in accord with reality, or if they possibly reflect some body-image distortion (see chapter 4).

● Do your clothes fit properly and look attractive on you? They might be tight because you have put on weight in the recent past. They might fit because you have acquired a large-size wardrobe. If the latter, are they attractive, and do they help improve your appearance?

● Do you like what you see when you look in the mirror?

● Can you undertake the physical activity you would like to? If you cannot, is excess weight a major factor?

Social Criteria

Social criteria combine objective and subjective elements; they are the possible social consequences of being overweight (see Appendixes A and B). These criteria exist because of the ways our society regards overweight people. Society's negative attitude is reflected back into how the overweight person feels, thinks, and acts. The following situations may exist for the overweight person, and may be used as criteria to help determine if he or she is too heavy:

● Diminished social life
● Diminished sex life
● Others making jokes, or worse, at the overweight person's expense
● Job discrimination

Criteria-Based Decision Making

To make your decision, you need to *feel* that you are too heavy. You need to say to yourself, I really don't like how I look in the mirror, and I'm going to do something about it that will work over the long haul. Or, It is wrong for people to discriminate against me because of my weight, but it is easier for me to change than to change them. So, I'm going to lose some weight. If you are like almost all successful weight-losers the subjective criteria will count the most for you in determining whether or not you are too heavy—that is, whether you are heavy enough that you really want to do something about it. For some people, 10 pounds above the upper limit for normal weight is too much; for others, 100 pounds over normal weight is perfectly acceptable.

Few successful weight-losers are motivated solely by objective criteria. For example, few people wake up one day, go to the BMI table (Table 2.1), determine that their BMI is 35, and then say, "It's time to lose weight." But the objective criteria are important. Although few people lose weight at age 30 because doing so will decrease their risk of heart disease at age 70, the risk reduction can be an important secondary motivator. In any case, the risk reduction is a side benefit to the most important benefits: feeling good physically and emotionally about yourself.

From the Take Control of Your Weight point of view, it is best if you use both objective and subjective criteria to make your decision.

What Now?

Once you have established intermediate objectives and an ultimate goal, you will probably find that designing your own Take Control program, and then carrying it out, will be easier than any of your previous weight-loss experiences.

3

Pathways to Weight Loss

What Is a Diet?

Although it is much less common today, in the past it was customary for weight-loss programs to be described as "diets." But diet has more than one meaning. It is also used to describe the sum total of foods we eat regularly. For example, a health professional is referring to that sum total when asking a patient, "What does your diet consist of?" Nutritionists and dieticians use the word to describe a wide variety of eating plans that help the body deal with certain diseases and negative health conditions. For example, special diets are recommended for managing ulcers, diabetes, high blood pressure, and high serum cholesterol.

Of course, the word *diet* is widely used in the world of weight loss, usually referring to some sort of calorie-restriction eating plan. We say, "I'm dieting," or "I'm on my diet," or "I'm going to start my diet next week." In this context it usually means a temporary, short-term, time-limited, and often quite rigid eating plan that will be in place only until a certain amount of weight is lost. Such a plan may or may not suggest permanent changes in the list of foods you eat regularly.

Time-limited weight-loss diets can be very specific in telling you what foods to eat at each meal, and how large the portion of each should be, for the period of time you will remain on the diet. Although calorie counting has dropped out of favor in recent years, replaced too often by a similarly austere commitment to fat-gram counting, it has long occupied a central place in many weight-loss diets. Calorie-counting diets usually offer specific menus for breakfast, lunch, and dinner, which keeps the caloric total of all food consumed for the day within a certain limit. They promise that if you follow the diet over a fixed number of days or weeks, you could expect to lose a given number of pounds.

Dieting and the Take Control of Your Weight Program

The Take Control of Your Weight Program does not include a diet in the conventional weight-loss sense. It does not offer calorie-counting or fat-gram counting menus or diet plans. However important changing your eating patterns may be to achieving success in weight loss, what you must do is achieve *permanent change* in your eating patterns. You should know and accept at this point that changing these patterns temporarily cannot help you in the long run, and might even hurt you. Thus, the Take Control of Your Weight Eating Plan aims at helping you to change your daily eating patterns by altering the list of foods from which you choose your meals.

Although calorie restriction is important for dealing with certain types of overweight, calorie counting, for practical reasons, will help few people change the way they eat permanently. How many people do you know who lost weight by actually counting calories every day, using either a chart or an electronic calculator? It's hard enough to do that for a week or two. Consider a lifetime of consulting a chart or calculator to determine what you will be eating for your next meal. The same reasoning applies to counting fat grams. Few people will spend their lives adding up the grams of fat they eat during a day, so they can know when they've reached their daily maximum.

On the other hand, what can work for you is making consciously *qualitative,* not consciously *quantitative,* decisions about your diet that result in changing the kinds of foods you eat instead of counting calories or fat grams. Over time, the qualitative changes will lead to a quantitative change in caloric intake that will happen in the natural course of events, not as the result of focusing on calorie or fat counts.

To be sure, the central element of the Take Control Eating Plan is reducing the amount of fat consumed. For health reasons, reducing the consumption of fatty foods is a wise course of action for all people, whether or not they want to lose weight. Doctors once believed that a diet that drew about 40 percent of its calories from fat was okay; now they know this percentage is much too high. The American Heart Association suggests the upper limit is 30 percent, but many nutritionists hold that the percentage should be even lower.

The way to achieve reduction in fat consumption is not through counting grams of fat, but by identifying the foods in your diet that are high in fat and gradually replacing them with appealing low-fat foods. Chapter 5 covers this process in detail. The Take Control Eating Plan provides lists of high-, medium-, and low-fat foods. You will be able to identify easily the foods that should go. And you will be able to find enough appealing foods in the medium- and low-fat categories to make the qualitative changes you need to make in your diet. If you are interested in foods that are not on the lists provided in this book, you *will* need a fat-gram counter to determine whether you should slowly add or eliminate those foods.

The Take Control Eating Plan offers no menus or diet plans. Why? Few people will be able to go through life following breakfast, lunch, and dinner menus provided by other people. In any case, making your own food choices is half the fun of eating. You should not have to decide between foods you are directed to eat and those you prefer to eat. Instead, you should concentrate your energy on the pleasure you expect from eating healthful and delicious foods.

Over time, healthy, delicious, low-fat foods will assume permanent places on the menu of your mind, just as your present high-fat diet (if it is high in fat) is on the present menu of your mind. The best way to imprint this new menu permanently in your consciousness is to create it yourself, over time, out of the low-fat foods you like best. This is what you will be doing as you develop and implement your own Take Control Eating Plan. After a while low-fat eating will be as natural for you as high-fat eating is for so many other Americans.

Benefits of Low-Fat Eating

Low-fat eating has many benefits. Let's review them briefly:

• Fats have more than twice the calories per gram than carbohydrates and proteins; therefore, they make a large contribution to creating and maintaining excess body weight.

• Eating foods high in fat, especially saturated fat, leads to elevated levels of cholesterol in the blood. High cholesterol levels (above 200 milligrams [mg] per deciliter [dl]) cause increased atherosclerosis, the accumulation of a layer of fatty substances on the inside walls of the arteries, which narrows the blood vessels that carry blood from your heart and lungs to your muscles, nerves, bones, and other body tissues and organs, including the heart. This narrowing of the coronary arteries causes heart attacks. Thus, an elevated blood cholesterol level, directly related to high dietary fat and cholesterol intake, causes an increased risk of cardiovascular disease.

In describing food fats, the word *saturated* refers to the chemical structure of certain kinds of fats. There are also unsaturated fats of two kinds, poly- and mono-. These fats, found in foods such as sesame, cottonseed, corn, sunflower, safflower, and soybean oils (*poly*unsaturated) and olive, canola, peanut, avocado, and nut oils (*mono*unsaturated), tend to lower blood cholesterol levels. Although unsaturated fats are not related to cholesterol problems, all kinds of fats are high in calories, and for this reason even they should be restricted in the diet.

   • High dietary fat intake has been associated with increased risk of cancers of the colon and prostate, although evidence does not support causal linkages to these diseases as well as it supports linkages to cardiovascular disease. A reduction of dietary fat may reduce the risk for all these diseases.

   If high dietary fat does indeed cause increased cancer risk, it may do so in three ways: (1) as a direct promoter of cancer; (2) as a cause of obesity, which is associated with increased cancer risk; and (3) by displacing foods in one's diet that are thought to decrease cancer risk, such as certain fruits (citrus, strawberries, and melons), vegetables (broccoli and other members of the cabbage family), and whole grains.

Common Problems of Eating and Exercise

There are a number of problems commonly related to eating and exercise. It is likely that you will have to deal with one or more of them if you are to be a successful weight-loser. Five eating problems are commonly known to contribute to overweight:

   • Too much fat in the diet
   • Too much sugar and other simple carbohydrates
   • Inconsistency in food choices over time
   • Skipping meals, with subsequent catching up
   • Eating three fairly healthy meals but then adding a fourth meal, usually a midnight snack

Few overweight people have all five of the above eating problems. But most overweight people have at least two of them, though seldom in equal measure. The Take Control Eating Plan will help you to identify which of the problems you have and show you how to handle them. Recall, however, that there are some people with LCO (low-calorie overweight), who may show none of these destructive habits. They eat properly and still cannot lose weight. The Take Control program has something to offer them too, as we shall discuss later.

Exercise

Several common problems related to exercise are shared by many overweight people, and indeed by many people who don't consider themselves overweight. Should you want or need to exercise regularly, you will probably have to deal with one or more of these problems.

The most common problem is, of course, not exercising at all, having a sedentary life-style—in popular speech, being a couch potato.

Another common problem is exercising not regularly but in fits and starts. This problem is generally characterized by two patterns. In the first, the frequency of exercise is the problem, even though the commitment may continue over a long period of time. For example, a person might work out intensively once a week or once every second week, and stay with this pattern for many months at a time. The second pattern involves a regular exercise regimen that is carried out irregularly. Here, a person might exercise three or four times a week, follow the schedule religiously for three months, and then, for some reason—an illness, extended travel, a lot of work, family activities around the holidays—abandon the schedule, only to resume it several months later and restart the cycle. Neither of these patterns is helpful to the body.

Then there is the overly enthusiastic convert. Though you haven't done anything for a very long time, for some reason you suddenly get caught up in an exercise fervor. This time you convince yourself that you are really going to get into it. The very first day, you run five miles, at your best clip, or you do an hour of high-impact aerobics, or, at age 38 you start weight lifting at a level close to what you were doing in high school. The next morning you hurt so much all over that you can barely get out of bed. You have no choice but to back off to let the pain subside, but by the time your body is again ready, the fervor may very well have left you. Conversely, you may grit your teeth and continue at the same level of intensity, deciding to see your way through the pain. This approach commonly leads to injury, which also leads to the end of the exercise program.

Finally, there is the Not Fun problem. Whatever exercise you choose, however you go about it, you just don't enjoy your exercise. And if you get no pleasure out of it, you are not going to do it regularly, no matter how dedicated you are. If you are to become a regular exerciser, it is imperative that you find an exercise program that you can enjoy.

The Take Control Exercise Plan will help you to deal with these common problems that deter so many people from exercising regularly.

Dealing with the Problems

Standard Interventions

All weight-loss programs must address the problems of eating and exercise. They usually do so by employing one or more of the following three kinds of psychological intervention: *behavioral, cognitive,* and *psychodynamic.* At times you might see a fourth intervention included—appetite-suppressant drugs—or even a fifth—surgery—but these are not, and should not be, available other than as part of a physician-supervised attempt to manage a body weight situation that has a clear pathological aspect to it.

Sometimes you will encounter a program that states that it employs weight-loss *methods* including "calorie restriction, exercise, behavior modification, and appetite-suppressant drugs." However, these four elements are not of the same order. As noted, the *use* of behavioral modification and appetite-suppressant drugs are not ends in themselves. They are methods and interventions *used to achieve* calorie restriction or some other change in your eating patterns, or *to cause* you to exercise regularly. Eating pattern changes and regular exercise are used to achieve weight loss, but interventions such as behavioral modification are what you *do* to affect your eating and physical activity. Such interventions are not the altered eating or exercise patterns themselves.

The Take Control of Your Weight Program includes major elements of each of the following standard interventions. As you go through the program, you will learn to recognize them when they appear.

Behavioral modification. Behavior mod, as it is called, is the most common intervention used by weight-loss programs. It is designed to effect action by affecting thinking. Although behavioral modification recognizes that thoughts and feelings exist, it directly addresses action and attempts to alter or break destructive patterns of behavior without concern for the attitudes or problems that established the patterns. This approach helps you reach your desired goal without having to understand the biochemical, physiological, or psychological factors in either weight gain or weight loss.

You may be familiar with the kinds of behaviors encouraged: eating only three meals a day, putting smaller portions on your plate, refusing second helpings, buying only healthy foods at the supermarket, chewing each bite for a longer time, eating more slowly, and so forth. Behavioral modification can be helpful not only for reducing caloric intake, but also for lowering the fat in your diet. We shall discuss it in some detail in chapter 5.

The cognitive approach. This intervention attempts to give you an intellectual understanding of the biochemical, physiological, and psychological factors influencing weight gain and loss. The theory is that if you know why you gained weight and understand the science behind your chosen weight-loss method, you will significantly increase your chances of success. The cognitive approach assumes that distortions (misunderstandings) in your thought processes contributed to your weight gain. It postulates that if the knowledge gaps are filled in, your future behavior will change for the better.

The psychodynamic approach. This approach examines the underlying psychological causes of overweight in some people: lack of approval in childhood, the use of food by parents as a reward for good behavior, low self-esteem, fear of sex or relationships, distorted body image, fear of failure, fear of success, and so forth. The assumption and hope are that the psychological forces behind destructive behavior will be devitalized if the dysfunctional processes can be identified. A person who has a clear understanding of what can or should be done to correct destructive behavior will have a better chance of guiding his or her future behavior.

Changing Habits

Human beings are creatures of habit. Two incontrovertible facts of human behavior as it relates to habit are relevant to the weight-loss process. First, the longer you have had a habit, the more difficult it is for you to abandon it. Second, changing a habit, especially a long-standing one, is always disquieting. You develop habits to spare yourself the anxiety of making all those decisions about what you are going to do next. Therefore, the more aggressively you try to change a habit, the more ill at ease you become, and the more strongly your psyche tries to push you back into the familiar and secure comfort of the old habit.

As the Take Control program will show you, there is no single, earth-shaking step to take, either in eating or exercise, that is going to change your life. Instead, you will embark on a series of small, easy steps, none of which by themselves will seriously threaten you but which together will over time transform the way you eat and expend energy in very significant ways. *Gradual change is the key to permanent changes.*

Are you currently eating a rather high-fat diet? You will not be told that from this day forward you will be forever denied fat in your diet. Nor will you be told to get all the fat out of your diet by next week or the week after. You will not be required to eliminate all the butter, chocolate, ice cream, and red meat by the end of the month.

Instead, you will choose one class of fatty food, and work to reduce or eliminate it. Are you eating ice cream four times a week? Well, next week eat it three times, and do that for two weeks. Then twice a week for two weeks, and so forth. Simultaneously, you will gradually substitute some other food for one you are trying to ease out of your diet, perhaps ice milk or low- or no-fat yogurt for ice cream (see chapter 5).

The same approach will apply in changing exercise habits. If you do not exercise at all, you will not start out by joining a gym or running four miles four times a week. You will set an intermediate objective for yourself of being able to walk, just plain walk, for 10 minutes, three times a week. By reaching this intermediate objective, you will have begun to deal with the hardest part of a regular exercise program, that is, the regularity (see chapter 7).

You can see that gradual change combines elements of the behavioral, cognitive, and psychodynamic approaches. For example, you are beginning to do certain things, and the repetition of your actions (practiced behavior) makes it more likely you will continue doing these same things in the future. But you are also giving yourself a chance, over a reasonable period of time, to marshal your newly acquired understanding of metabolism to help you accept, believe in, and welcome your new way of life. Psychologically, you will deal with certain paralyzing, inhibiting fears, such as the fear of change or the fear of failure. By making gradual one-small-step-at-a-time changes, disruption of your old ways will present a less frightening scenario. Because gradual change is the best way to make your psyche accept change, it may be the only way to make change stick.

There are no shortcuts to weight loss, particularly for the person with diet-induced low-calorie overweight. In fact, as you by now know, trying easy shortcuts causes diet-induced low-calorie overweight. Gradual change is the easiest way to lose weight. No big leaps forward mean no long falls backward. It's the painless way to change your eating habits. It's the gentle way to become a regular exerciser.

The Three Pathways Down

Depending on which of the four Pathways Up you took to overweight (see pages 23–24), you will have to do one or more of the following in order to lose weight:

- Reduce total caloric intake.
- Lower the amount of fat in your diet as a means of lowering caloric intake.

• Engage in regular exercise as a way to burn up excess calories stored in body fat and as a way to raise your resting metabolic rate.

By considering the three elements above and the nature of the four Pathways Up, we have determined that there are three possible Pathways Down—A, B, and C:

A. Reducing caloric intake obligatory, regular exercise desirable
B. Reducing caloric intake and regular exercise both equally important
C. Regular exercise obligatory, low-fat eating desirable, with some overall reduction in caloric intake not a goal but a likely consequence

Chapter 4 presents greater detail about how you can match the correct Pathway Down to your Pathway Up. At this point, you should be able to see that if your overweight is caused by overeating, Pathway A is the choice down for you. If you have family-induced overweight, Pathway B is the one you will want to follow down. Finally, if you have either genetically predisposed or diet-induced low-calorie overweight, Pathway C should work best for you.

Pathway C and the Take Control Eating Plan. If you are on Pathway C, your most important concern should be regular exercise. However, there are several reasons why you should also follow the Take Control Eating Plan.

• As regular exercise raises your resting metabolic rate (RMR), you want to make sure that you keep your caloric intake down, so that your body will use its stored fat to meet the higher energy need. The easiest way to assure this, without counting calories, is through low-fat eating.

• If you eat food containing more calories than your body requires to meet its energy needs, make sure that the extra calories are in the form of carbohydrates or proteins. The body rapidly converts food fat to body fat, but it has much more difficulty converting carbohydrates and proteins to body fat.

• Some studies suggest that in order to process food fat for energy, the body must first convert a considerable part of the food fat to body fat. Thus a diet having most of its caloric value in fat, rather than carbohydrate or protein, seems to assure a continued buildup of stored body fat.

• Even if you use exercise as the primary vehicle to reach a preferred body weight, you should get into the habit of healthy, low-fat eating so that any interruption of your exercise program will not result in a sudden increase in your weight.

• Many people find that they feel better when they reduce the amount of fat in their diet. Many report a heavy feeling after eating a high-fat meal. If you eat a high-fat meal or snack late at night, you may find yourself waking in the morning to such a heavy feeling that you have difficulty getting started for the day ahead.

4

Overweight and You:

Self-Assessment

IT IS IMPORTANT to remember that overweight is not a disease. At moderate levels it is a condition considered by some people to be unsightly, uncomfortable, and/or counterproductive. Moderate obesity is also a risk factor for certain diseases, including hypertension, diabetes, and gall bladder disease. Uncommonly, the overweight condition is the result of some present disease, such as hypothyroidism or adrenal overactivity (Cushing's disease). At the highest weight levels, a condition called morbid obesity, there are direct effects on the lungs and heart, often leading to heart failure.

It is a fundamental error to presume that the underlying cause of obesity in all overweight people is the same simply because the common characteristic of obesity, in most cases high body weight, is identical in all overweight people. This presumption misses the important point that a person may have taken several possible Pathways Up to overweight, each quite different from the others. A major premise of the Take Control of Your Weight Program is that to achieve success, a person interested in losing weight must be able to distinguish among the causes of overweight. Each cause requires a different response to achieve success.

Assessing Your Health

Before you determine which Pathway Up you took to overweight, you should consider whether or not you need to be examined by a physician or other health professional to find out if your overweight condition is either a cause or a sign of disease requiring medical management. There are relatively few diseases for which overweight is a symptom. Nevertheless, some of these conditions are serious, and you should make sure you do not suffer from any of them.

   If you answer yes to any of the following questions, it would be a good idea to consult your doctor.

1. Do you have dry skin or dry/very fine hair?   Yes_____ No_____

2. Are you particularly uncomfortable in the cold? Do
   you have poor circulation?   Yes_____ No_____

3. Do you have a slow pulse? Are you dizzy or
   lightheaded, especially on standing or arising from
   bed?   Yes_____ No_____

4. Do you find that you are fatigued or lethargic much
   of the time, or that you still feel tired after eight
   hours of sleep?   Yes_____ No_____

5. Are you constipated, bloated, or crampy?   Yes_____ No_____

6. Do you get short of breath easily? Does fluid ever
   collect in your legs? Do you get pain in your chest,
   jaw, or arms if you get very anxious, after you eat,
   or on exertion?   Yes_____ No_____

7. Do you frequently suffer from headaches?   Yes_____ No_____

8. Do you sleep poorly, have a poor memory, or have
   difficulty concentrating?   Yes_____ No_____

9. Do you have red or purplish stretch marks? Are
   your arms and legs thin compared to your body?   Yes_____ No_____

If you answered yes to one or more of these questions, don't panic. Many of the symptoms listed above are what doctors call nonspecific, meaning that they can have more than one underlying cause. Still, a yes answer to any of these questions should cause you to make an appointment with your family doctor to discuss those signs and symptoms you believe you have, not only in relation to your weight problem but also to determine whether or not you are suffering from some other malady of which you may be unaware. Once a diagnosis has been made and, if necessary, a treatment plan for the disease instituted, you can discuss with your doctor the advisability of your starting on a weight-reduction plan.

   If you did not answer yes to any of the above questions and feel you are in good health generally, changing your eating habits or becoming a regular exerciser should present little risk to your health—provided you follow the guidelines for gradual change. However, if you have ever been diagnosed as having a disease or condition for which exercise might be contraindicated, it would be a good idea to get a medical checkup and your physician's clearance before beginning the Take Control program. Do any of the statements on the following list apply to you?

1. You have been found to have high blood pressure.
2. You have been told you have high blood cholesterol.
3. You have been diagnosed as having cardiovascular disease.
4. You have a history of lung problems.
5. You use prescribed medication on a regular basis.
6. You are a cigarette smoker or you engage in excessive use of drugs or alcohol.
7. You have bone or joint problems.
8. You have been diagnosed as having a chronic illness such as diabetes.

If any of the statements in the above list apply to you, regular exercise under medical supervision could be a major aid in managing many of them. If you take medication for borderline hypertension, for example, your doctor may find that after you have been on a regular exercise program for a period of time your blood pressure will have dropped sufficiently to allow him or her to recommend a trial period off the medication. Regular exercise has also been shown to reduce cholesterol levels, and to raise the HDL (high density lipoprotein), a fraction of your total cholesterol that protects against heart disease. Monitoring your serum cholesterol levels as you get into a regular exercise program might give your doctor a good reason to try lowering or discontinuing any cholesterol-lowering medication you may now be taking.

Psychological History

The next series of questions concerns your general psychological status. As explained in Appendix B, most overweight people, like most other people, have some psychological problems.

Given its cost and the difficulty in finding therapists qualified to deal with weight-related problems, psychotherapy is neither indicated nor justified for most overweight people. Yet some overweight people are at some risk because of underlying psychological problems. Some weight problems can remain intractable without guidance on how psychological factors may be contributing to or exacerbating them.

If you answer yes to any of the first three questions below, or to more than

two or three of the others, you may want to consult a health professional with
education and experience in dealing with overweight as an expression of psychological problems.

1. Are you "clinically depressed"? Clinically depressed
   does not mean being unhappy or blue on occasion.
   We all go through that. It does mean that you are
   down *most of the time* and find it *very difficult* to
   work or go to school, or to carry out the other
   normal activities of life.   Yes_____   No_____

2. Is your self-concept based almost entirely on what
   you think your body looks like, or what you believe
   others think your body looks like?   Yes_____   No_____

3. Do you binge and purge, that is, overeating
   followed by self-induced vomiting or use of
   diuretics or laxatives?   Yes_____   No_____

4. Do you live in the "future conditional"? That is, do
   you tend to put your life on hold until after the diet
   you are currently on has been completed, which
   would make the gradual-change approach
   especially difficult for you?   Yes_____   No_____

5. Do you have an overall sense that food-related
   decisions dominate your life, that the question of
   whether or not to eat and what to eat preoccupies
   you, that your body and its fat seem to be primarily
   responsible for any unhappiness you feel about
   your life?   Yes_____   No_____

6. Is feeling guilty a very important and frequently felt
   factor in your dieting/not dieting behavior?   Yes_____   No_____

7. Do you very easily and frequently become angry,
   frustrated, or feel loss of control over issues of
   eating?   Yes_____   No_____

8. Do you find that you are very often taken over by
   feelings either of failure or susceptibility to
   temptation?   Yes_____   No_____

9. Do you believe that dietary restraint and eternal
   vigilance are required at all times in order to control
   your weight, to the extent that the subject
   dominates your thoughts about eating and food?   Yes____   No____

Remember that a certain amount of preoccupation with weight is inevitable, given the values of our society. Consequently, you may have hesitated before answering one or two of the above questions. However, even a thought that one of the first three questions might describe your own situation should lead you to seek qualified and competent professional help.

How to Find a Qualified Professional

If you decide to seek professional help, you should bear in mind that not every psychotherapist is a licensed practitioner, that not every person identified as a nutritionist has the academic training to support the designation, and that the counselor in your local weight-loss center may have had no training beyond how to sell you a contract.

Unfortunately, many fully licensed and credentialed health practitioners know little about overweight and the psychological problems associated with it. Very few practicing physicians have received any training in nutrition, and even fewer are educated about weight loss. Too many physicians, especially those whose medical education took place many years ago, still consider overweight a condition brought on solely by the patient's self-indulgence, and therefore curable with willpower. It is not surprising that physicians with this attitude are reluctant to devote valuable time to the study of the underlying physical or psychological causes of overweight.

Finally, even licensed professionals with competent training can—for reasons unrelated to you or your condition—recommend interventions that don't work very well, are simply not right for you, or may be unsafe in certain cases.

Still, you should not be discouraged. Many professionals are capable of helping you with your weight problem. Ask your friends who have sought similar help for names of people they found professional and competent. Ask your doctor to make inquiries for you about health professionals with current training in the field. Then personally check the credentials and educational background of the professionals whose names you have been given. (For example, you could go to your local library to consult the *Directory of Medical Specialists*.) As your list gets shorter, ask about the technical knowledge each person brings to his or her practice, ascertain if there may be some conflict of interest attached to the particular program each is recommending, and try to determine if what the person has to offer is suitable for dealing with your particular type of overweight or underlying problem.

Don't allow yourself to be intimidated by a professional's credentials or your relative ignorance of the field. You do not necessarily have to know precisely what a person is talking about in order to know if that person understands his or her subject. Evasive, impatient answers are sure signs that a professional's command of the material may not be complete. In general, if a professional cannot explain some aspect of the problem or solution so that an interested layperson can understand it, the chances are that the professional does not fully understand it.

If choosing the right person to help you distresses you to the extent that your problem is exacerbated by your increasing anxiety, you may need to ask a close friend or relative to aid you in your search. This friend or relative will not be involved in your therapy, but can accompany you on visits to potential therapists or other health practitioners and ask the hard questions that you might be afraid to ask for a variety of reasons.

The Take Control Self-Assessment Process

If your answers to the health status and psychological history questions lead you to believe you are ready to proceed with the Take Control program, move now to a series of questions about your personal weight history, your family history of overweight and related conditions, and your eating behavior and dieting history. Each section contains a guide to help you evaluate your answers.

Your answers should enable you to determine what Pathway Up you took. Knowing what kind of overweight you have will help you determine the correct Pathway Down to help you reach the weight level that you believe to be appropriate and achievable.

Physical Measures of Overweight

Most people engaged in weight loss use a weight-measuring scale, of course. It can be a blessing or a curse. We are happy when the numbers go down, unhappy when they go up. But it is really important that you not become a slave to the scale. In fact, the Take Control of Your Weight Program recommends that once you start the program you refrain from looking at your scale weight for at least two weeks, and preferably for four. Recall that this program focuses on gradual change and long-term success, avoiding the trap of seeking immediate gratification.

However, as part of your general self-assessment, you will have to take your weight before you start the program. This will provide one reference by which you can measure success as you follow your Pathway Down. Two other physical measures of overweight that go beyond simple scale weight are the waist-to-hip ratio (WHR) and the body mass index (BMI) (see chapter 2). You may want to determine either one or both before you start, so you can use the numbers for comparison purposes later on.

Finally, you must consider matters related to your self-image. What do you see when you look in the mirror? How do you honestly feel about yourself? Is your own evaluation of your overweight confirmed by the judgment of others who will tell you the truth? Do they see you as more overweight or less overweight than you see yourself?

Personal Weight History

The first set of questions to help you identify your Pathway Up focuses on an assessment of your weight.

1. How much do you weigh?
2. Look at Table I.1 (see page 9). Using the chart as a guideline, are you overweight? If you are, roughly how much do you believe is fat, how much muscle?
3. If you are overweight, how long have you been at your present weight?
4. Have you ever been thin? If you have never thought of yourself as thin, has your weight ever been within the normal weight range for you, according to Table I.1?
5. If you are currently overweight, how old were you when your weight was last in the normal range? What has been your minimum weight as an adult?
6. Are you now at your heaviest? If not, what was your highest weight as an adult?
7. If you have been at "normal" weight in the past, have one or more major life events preceded your weight gain? For example: puberty or the later teenage years, getting married, having a child, moving, getting separated or divorced, becoming a widow(er), changing your job or your career (or having to give it up for any reason).

The answers to these questions can help you think about the following issues.

Are you really overweight, in the physical sense? Or are you possibly like the magazine editor whose story is presented in Appendix B? At 5 feet 7 inches, 124 pounds, she actually felt herself to be "slightly heavy," though she could not have been overweight by any objective standard. If you are not physically overweight, have you considered that instead of trying to lose weight, you might perhaps be better off trying to deal with the issues making you think of yourself as fat?

Alternatively, after considering your answers to these questions, you may remain unhappy with your body shape despite the fact that your weight is within normal limits by accepted standards. You might then decide to begin a program of moderate exercise designed to build up your musculature and reduce body flabbiness, without concerning yourself with weight loss. If your goal is to improve your appearance and sense of well-being, exercise can do that in many cases, even in the absence of significant weight loss. And combining exercise with low-fat eating can bring you some positive changes in body appearance, as well as even stronger life-style and health benefits.

If you are truly overweight, how much would you have to lose to get your weight within the normal weight range for your height and frame? Will that make you happy, or do you really feel you will have to lose more? Is becoming really thin the only result that will please you? If so, why? Answering these questions honestly will be important in defining your goals for the program, as well as helping in your self-assessment.

If you haven't been overweight all of your life, identifying the point in your life cycle when the problem started will help you determine your Pathway Up. It will also help you deal with the question of how feasible it is for you to attempt weight loss: What are your chances of success? If you have always been heavy, you should be prepared for a more difficult (although not necessarily impossible) journey than if your weight was in the normal range into your late adolescent or adult years. These are also factors to consider when deciding how much weight you should try to lose.

Eating Behavior History

Your answers to the following questions will help you understand what your eating patterns really are, which is important in determining the changes you need to make in order to achieve your goals.

1. How much do you eat? Do you think of yourself as an undereater, a normal eater, or an overeater?
2. If you are an overeater or an undereater, have you always been that way? How has your eating level been connected with your weight-gain experience and your present weight state?
3. In general, what kind of food do you eat? The specifics of your food

selections will be discussed in chapter 5, but for now think about the types of food you eat. Do you tend to eat a lot of meat, a lot of fat? Do you frequently consume alcoholic beverages, especially beer? Do you like sweets, such as candy, cake, pie, and ice cream? Do you eat them often?

4. How many meals do you eat a day? One, two, three, four, or more? Do you frequently skip breakfast? Eat a very light lunch? Snack all evening or just before bedtime?

5. Do you find it hard to be certain if you are physically hungry? Or if you are full after you have eaten a certain amount?

6. Do you frequently eat for reasons other than physical hunger (e.g., unconscious nibbling, snacking because you are nervous or bored, overeating because it is holiday time)?

7. Are there other cues not related to hunger that make you eat (e.g., seeing a particular TV show or sports event on television, walking into the kitchen, seeing a full refrigerator, not wanting to waste food, knowing that there are cookies or rich crackers in the cupboard)?

You should know by now that how much and what kinds of food you eat tell you much about what kind of overweight you have. If you are an overeater (or have been one in the past, without converting to undereating in the interim), the chances are good that you have pure overeating overweight. If you are an overeater, starting to think about the kinds of foods you like to eat will help you begin planning for the necessary changes in your eating patterns.

Becoming conscious of the number of meals you eat each day can help you too. Some overeaters eat too much simply because they eat a fourth meal—the late-night snack just before bedtime. Some people have lost significant amounts of weight by eliminating the fourth meal.

If you answered yes to one or more of the questions that concern the role of hunger and other cues in your eating, you may be an excellent candidate for intervention using one or more behavioral techniques that are reviewed in chapter 5.

Family History

It is not always a simple matter to distinguish between family-induced and genetically predisposed overweight. After all, both run in families. But there are some significant differences, and the answers to the following questions can help you sort them out.

1. Are/were either/both of your parents overweight? For all of their lives? Or only part? Were their parents overweight?
2. Are/were any of your siblings overweight?
3. Were you heavy when you were a child?
4. What were the eating patterns you experienced in childhood? Did they match those described in chapter 1 in the section on family-induced overweight? In other words, were you brought up in a rich food, eat-eat-eat environment?
5. Do you have any relatives who are/were morbidly obese (i.e., more than 100 pounds overweight)? For all, or only part of their adult lives?
6. Does/did anyone in your immediate family have any of the following obesity-related medical conditions: diabetes, high blood pressure, high fat level in the blood (hyperlipidemia)?
7. Is there a cultural attitude in your family regarding desirable body size/shape?
8. In your family, are/were there any attitudes toward food and eating that you believe encouraged weight gain?
9. Was weight-loss dieting of various kinds common in your family when you were a child?

If you generally answered no to these questions, it is unlikely that you have either genetically predisposed or family-induced overweight. The relationship among the various combinations of yes answers is complex, and there is still much to learn about these two causes of overweight. But a few conclusions can safely be made.

If you were overweight as a child, your Pathway Up is probably family-induced or genetically predisposed. But the existence of overweight in childhood alone does not permit us to distinguish between the causes. Neither does the finding of simply having overweight parents. Also, genetic predisposition does not require the appearance of overweight in childhood.

The chances are good that you have family-induced overweight if you were overweight as a child, *and* your parents (and probably your siblings as well) were overweight, *and* food and eating were dealt with as described in chapter 1, *and* you are currently eating a high- or normal-calorie diet. If you have also engaged in sudden calorie-restrictive dieting, you could have diet-induced low-calorie overweight (LCO) superimposed upon family-induced overweight.

You probably have genetically predisposed LCO if one or both parents were overweight (and possibly your siblings as well), *and* food was *not* ample on the table during your childhood, *and* weight-loss dieting was common in your family, *and* you have had a lot of difficulty losing weight as an adult, *and* you have been eating a low-calorie diet for quite some time without achieving desired weight loss.

If you have genetically predisposed LCO, you may find it especially difficult to lose weight. You may have a built-in "biological limit." You may be genetically programmed to carry around more body fat than do many other people. If that is the case, you might choose to focus on lowering the fat in your diet and exercising regularly for health and life-style reasons and to build up muscle mass to change your appearance.

It also seems possible that some people may have diet-induced LCO imposed on top of genetically predisposed LCO, but much more research must be done before we can distinguish between the two types with any degree of certainty. However, as you will see in chapter 5, the approach to LCO is the same, regardless of its origins.

Dieting History

The following questions focus on diet-induced low-calorie overweight. If you immediately answer yes to more than half of these questions, it is very likely that diet-induced LCO is your Pathway Up.

1. Have you dieted so frequently that you could call yourself a chronic dieter?
2. Have you ever tried to lose weight on a fad diet (such as a fruit-only, grain-only, or high-protein diet)?
3. Have you ever tried unsuccessfully to lose weight on a low-calorie diet (fewer than 1,000 calories per day), liquid or otherwise?
4. Do you often cut back on your caloric intake to about 1,000 calories per day or fewer for short periods of time and remain overweight?
5. Is your regular intake fewer than 1,000 calories per day, but you remain overweight?
6. Have you successfully lost 10 pounds or more on a crash diet over a short period of time, two to three weeks, only to regain it within two to three months after you finished the diet?
7. Dieting as you have, have you experienced major fluctuations in your weight more than twice? Are you a "yo-yo" dieter?
8. Do you pay no attention to physical hunger when you are dieting?
9. Do you frequently starve yourself for a day, or longer?

10. Do you think of each diet as a short-term solution?
11. Do you think of each new diet as the last one you will ever have to use, the last remedy for your overweight problem?
12. Do you think that if you are not currently on a diet, you have blown it or are in a pigging-out stage?
13. Do you weigh more now than you did before you started dieting?

Diet-induced low-calorie overweight is probably the most common class of overweight in this country (see chapter 1). Despite a long history of failure, it can be dealt with successfully. However, doing so takes work and patience to change the pattern that has produced only failure.

How to Match Your Pathway Up with the Correct Pathway Down

Now that you probably know your Pathway Up, you need to consider the several available Pathways Down. The process of matching your Pathways Up and Down should be straightforward for you. The weight-loss tools from which you will fashion your program are (1) reduction of total caloric intake, (2) lowering the amount of fat in your diet, and (3) engaging in regular exercise. Combining these tools, you can create for yourself one of three possible Pathways Down:

A. Reducing caloric intake obligatory, regular exercise desirable
B. Reducing caloric intake and regular exercise both equally important
C. Regular exercise obligatory, low- or lower-fat eating desirable, with a reduction in caloric intake not a factor

Pathway A

If you have followed the *overeating* Pathway Up, Pathway A is the route Down for you. Unless you have diet-induced LCO superimposed upon your overeating behavior, it is likely that your resting metabolic rate (RMR) is in the normal range (see chapter 1). To lose weight you need to reduce your caloric intake and, if possible, increase your caloric expenditure. The Take Control Eating Plan will help you lower both the fat and the simple carbohydrates in your diet and, if necessary, cut back on your total intake. The role of regular exercise will be to help burn extra calories stored as body fat.

Pathway B

If you have followed the *family-induced* Pathway Up, Pathway B is the route Down for you. Again, unless you have diet-induced low-calorie overweight (LCO) superimposed, it is likely that your RMR is in the normal range. You need to reduce your caloric intake and increase your caloric expenditure. But since you are likely to have a normal caloric intake, it is important to guard against LCO as you follow any weight-loss program. To do so, you will cut back on your caloric intake primarily by reducing the fat in your diet. Regular exercise will burn extra calories and add protection against the development of diet-induced LCO.

Pathway C

If you have followed either the *genetically predisposed* or the *diet-induced LCO* Pathway Up, Pathway C is the route Down for you. Your resting metabolic rate (RMR) is depressed (see chapter 1). You are already eating a low-calorie diet and not losing weight. So more calorie restriction will only make the problem worse. The objective for you is to raise your RMR, and the only known way to do this is regular exercise.

The key to Pathway C is building up muscle mass. Muscle requires more energy per pound to keep it functioning, even when it is not used, than does body fat. As you lose weight, if you lose muscle as well as fat, your RMR will actually go down, even without stimulating the starvation response. You can end up requiring less food on a daily basis than you did before you started losing weight. On the other hand, if you exercise regularly, you will slowly and gradually build up your muscle mass, thus raising your RMR. As your RMR is brought closer to normal, you will begin drawing energy from your stored body fat. You will gradually lose weight, assuming that you don't increase your caloric intake to match the new levels of energy consumption.

An important point about exercise and its role in raising the RMR is that we are not necessarily talking about weight lifting or any other very vigorous exercise. *Any regular exercise will increase muscle mass.* Some routines will do it faster and to a greater extent, but *all* will do it. We will discuss regular exercise in detail in chapters 7 through 9.

Reducing the amount of fat consumed is also recommended for LCO, but a reduction in fat intake alone will not help you lose weight. If you have genetically predisposed or diet-induced low-calorie overweight, you will have to become a regular exerciser to lose weight. It sounds simple enough, but for some people it is not an easy task.

Exercise: Physicians' Attitudes

In past days, doctors tended to dismiss the value of exercise in weight reduction because they considered only the calories expended during the period of exercise itself. Many patients were told that they would have to walk 36 miles to lose one pound; others were told with a chuckle that the only useful exercise was to place your palms firmly against the edge of the dining-room table and push. Even today, few physicians seem to know very much about exercise, and until recently the medical profession shied away from recommending exercise for patients. You may even run into a physician who still tells his or her patients that regular exercise is not good for them, might even harm them, or has little if anything to do with weight loss.

Perhaps part of the reason for this lack of interest in exercise is that many physicians do not feel in control of this kind of therapy. If they prescribe two tablets of a medication four times a day, they can reasonably expect that you will take the prescribed dose at the prescribed times. But many doctors feel they cannot be confident that their prescription to walk for 30 minutes a day will be observed as faithfully, so they often fail to use exercise as a part of treatment. This is counterproductive, for exercise is the very best prescription for many kinds of overweight and for many types of conditions for which drugs are now routinely prescribed.

If you are not satisfied with your physician's level of knowledge and attitude about exercise, try another doctor. Physician-run cardiofitness or sports medicine centers are good places to go if you cannot get the help you need from your own practitioner.

5

Healthy Eating

THERE ARE THREE principal reasons why this first chapter about the Take Control Eating Plan is entitled "Healthy Eating" instead of something like "Eating for Weight Loss."

The first reason, of course, is that success in weight loss should be defined not only by how much weight you lose, but also by whether or not you can maintain your target weight over time.

Second, if calorie restriction is a major element of your particular Pathway Down, the best, easiest, and healthiest way to achieve that calorie restriction is *not* by focusing on the calorie content of everything you eat. Instead, a simple, gradual, reduction in the amount of fat in your regular diet works best. As mentioned previously, fat contains more than twice the number of calories, gram for gram, as carbohydrate or protein, and because the body stores consumed fat as body fat much more efficiently than it converts carbohydrate or protein to body fat for storage.

Third, as virtually all studies show, healthy eating should be a goal of all people, whether or not they see themselves as overweight. Low-fat eating can reduce the risk of developing many serious diseases. Healthy diets contain many nutritional elements, such as dietary fiber, that should be consumed on a regular basis by all people. Some of our most beneficial foods, shown in study after study to contribute to good health, are often crowded out by the "siren foods," those high in sugar and fat.

First Thoughts

Before you can begin extracting and using the ideas that can be most helpful to you, you must decide which Pathway Down you want to pursue in your quest for a healthier life. Recall the three possible Pathways Down:

A. Reducing caloric intake obligatory, regular exercise desirable
B. Reducing caloric intake and regular exercise both equally important
C. Regular exercise obligatory, low-fat eating desirable.

If your correct Pathway Down is A or B, the Take Control Eating Plan is a must for you. However, even if your correct Pathway Down is C, in which low-fat eating is desirable though not obligatory, the Take Control Eating Plan can provide valuable benefits for you (see chapter 3 and Appendix A).

Finally, you may have decided that weight loss will prove very difficult if not impossible for you, but you want to eat right to be healthier and to feel better. Obviously, low-fat eating is for you.

What Is Healthy Eating?

The principles of healthy eating are presented in the *Dietary Guidelines for Americans*, published as a joint effort by the U.S. Department of Agriculture and Department of Health and Human Services (see Chart 5.1):

- Eat a variety of foods.
- Maintain a healthy weight.
- Choose a diet low in fat, saturated fat, and cholesterol.
- Use sugars only in moderation.
- Use salt only in moderation.
- If you drink alcoholic beverages, do so in moderation.

This list specifies eating behaviors that should lead to and protect good health in all people, not just those who are overweight. Note that it also suggests a low-fat diet, especially one low in saturated fat. Variety and balance come from choosing among the five food groups. You may remember the old Basic Four Food Groups; now there are five. Also, eating from each of the five groups in roughly equivalent proportions—as we once ate from the old Basic Four—is no longer advised.

The Food Guide Pyramid, published in 1992 as part of the newest version of *Dietary Guidelines for Americans,* also has a sixth category—Fats, Oils, & Sweets. This sixth category is offered not as a food group from which we should draw nutritional benefits but only as a concession to reality, in that people eat these foods. Since they contribute little to health, the recommendation is that we should eat them sparingly.

The new Food Guide Pyramid recommends that 2 to 3 servings should be taken daily from the milk products group and the same number of servings daily from the meat group. The fruit group should provide 2 to 4 servings and the vegetable group 3 to 5. The bread, cereal, rice, and pasta group should provide a whopping 6 to 11 servings daily. Clearly, eating roughly equivalent amounts of food from each group is no longer recommended.

The American Heart Association establishes the following as typical adult-size servings:

- Fruit: ½ cup fruit juice, one medium-size piece of fruit
- Vegetable: ½ cup vegetable juice, ½ to 1 cup of cooked or raw (nonstarchy) vegetable, ¼ to ½ cup of starchy vegetable
- Bread, etc.: one slice bread or tortilla; 1 cup dry flaked cereal, or ½ cup

CHART 5.1 *Food Guide Pyramid: A Guide to Daily Food Choice*

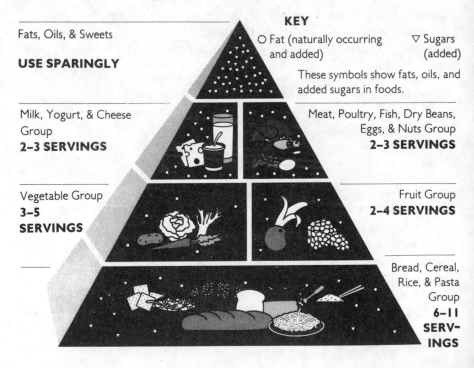

TABLE **5.1** *Calories and Fat Grams*
Daily Diet Supplying 30 Percent of Calories as Total Fat,
10 Percent as Saturated Fat

Total Calories Per Day	Total Fat Calories Per Day	Total Grams of Fat Per Day	Total Saturated Fat Calories Per Day	Total Grams of Saturated Fat Per Day
1,000	300	33	100	11
1,200	360	40	120	13
1,400	420	46	140	15
1,600	480	53	160	18
1,800	540	60	180	20
2,000	600	66	200	22
2,200	660	73	220	24
2,400	720	80	240	26
2,600	780	86	260	29
2,800	840	93	280	31
3,000	900	100	300	33
3,200	960	106	320	35
3,400	1,020	113	340	38
3,600	1,080	120	360	40

cooked cereal, or ¼ cup nugget- or bud-type cereal; 1 cup pasta, rice, or noodles; 2 graham crackers; 1 cup dry popcorn

• Milk, etc.: one 8-ounce glass of milk, 1 ounce cheese, ½ cup cottage cheese, 8 ounces yogurt

• Meat, etc.: 2 to 3 ounces cooked meat, fish, or poultry; 1 cup cooked beans, peas, or lentils; 3 ounces soybean curd (tofu)

• Fats, etc.: 1 teaspoon vegetable oil or margarine; 2 teaspoons diet margarine; 2 teaspoons salad dressing, mayonnaise, or peanut butter; 3 teaspoons seeds, nuts, chopped avocado, or olives.

What You Don't Do in the Take Control Program

You don't count calories and you don't count fat grams in the Take Control of Your Weight Program. For one thing, this attaches undesirable guilt feelings to a new way of eating. And there is a practical reason for controlling your fat and calorie intake *qualitatively* rather than *quantitatively*: Most people can't, don't, and won't count calories or fat grams forever. Therefore, the Take Control Eating Plan focuses on qualitative changes. Over time, sound qualitative changes in the way you eat will lead inevitably to quantitative change. This will happen gradually and naturally, not as the result of pressure to remain within strict calorie limits set by others.

What You Now Eat

Analyzing what and how you now eat is the first step in developing your own Take Control of Your Weight Eating Plan. The following sample eating log is that of a person we call Toby, someone who might read this book. To simplify our presentation, we have created Toby's eating log so that it illustrates each of the five major eating problems that contribute to overweight: too much dietary fat, too much sugar and other simple carbohydrates, inconsistency in food choices, skipping meals with subsequent catching up, and eating a fourth meal.

Toby's Eating Log

Day of Week	Breakfast	Lunch	Afternoon Snack	Dinner	Evening Snack
Mon.	Sugar cereal w/ whole milk Eng. muffin w/butter Coffee	Cheeseburg. Fr. fries Soda	Coffee w/ cream Cookies	Broiled chicken Baked pot. w/marg. Broccoli Fudge cake	Potato chips Diet soda
Tues.	Oat cereal w/2% milk Toast w/ marg. and jam Juice	None	Jelly beans, handful	Meatloaf w/gravy Mashed pot. w/ butter Salad w/ light dressing	Fudge cake Whole milk

Day of Week	Breakfast	Lunch	Afternoon Snack	Dinner	Evening Snack
Wed.	None	Pita bread Plain low-fat yogurt	Candy bar	Broiled fish Fr. fries Str. beans Flavored gelatin	Flavored gelatin w/ whipped cream
Thurs.	Scrambled eggs Bacon Toast w/ margarine Coffee w/ cream	Melted cheese sand. Corn chips Diet soda	None	Pork chops Salad w/ light dressing Str. beans w/butter sauce Ice cream	Ice cream
Fri.	Fresh fruit Oat bran muffin Coffee w/ nonfat creamer	Tuna in water Crisp bread Flavored seltzer	Decaf. w/ nonfat creamer Gingersnaps	Vegetarian dinner Melon Diet soda	None
Sat.	Cereal Fruit Coffee Juice	Fast food w/kids	Candy bar	Steak w/ pot. & veg. Fruit pie w/ ice cream	Popcorn w/butter, at the movies
Sun.	Pancakes w/butter & syrup Juice	Fast food w/kids	Apple	Chinese, out, w/ribs, egg roll, fried shrimp, fried rice	None

After looking at the log, it's probably safe to say that Toby's Pathway Up was pure overeating. Toby eats quite a lot of fat: butter, whole milk, cheese, cream in coffee, ice cream, fried foods, potato chips, red meat, candy bars. Toby also eats plenty of simple sugars: candy bars, sugared cereals, cake, ice cream. Toby's sample eating log also demonstrates an inconsistency in food choices, a common problem in the overweight person. Even when not on a diet, overweight people will often eat some foods that are frequently found on calorie-restriction diets.

On Monday, Toby eats three meals and two snacks, all brimming with fat and sugar. On Tuesday, a diet pang presents itself. The day begins with a healthy breakfast, followed by a skipped lunch, apparently with the thought that doing so will "help make up for yesterday" (it won't). But then hunger appears in midafternoon and a handful of jelly beans disappears from the bowl in the office. This simple sugar meal satisfies Toby's hunger only temporarily. Dinner is rather fatty, except for the counterpoint of low-oil salad dressing. It's all blown completely before bedtime—in the fridge there's some leftover fudge cake from yesterday. That yummy dish is washed down with a glass of whole milk.

On Wednesday, Toby wakes up with an overfull feeling from the fudge cake and milk. Today it's breakfast that's skipped. Toby manages to eat a "dietary lunch" taken from one of the low-cal wonder diets he used in the past. But again, the imbalance of this approach catches up with Toby, and he eats a candy bar for a snack. Nevertheless, determined not to let yesterday's pattern repeat itself, Toby has a healthy dinner. For nighttime snack, there is some leftover gelatin but because "pretty good" eating has been the order of the day, some whipped cream from the aerosol can in the fridge makes its way onto the gelatin.

Thursday is a high-fat day, with no attempt at any kind of dieting. Friday is just the reverse. Toby does know the components of a healthy diet, and tries to use them. But on the weekend, everything falls apart. High fat, high simple sugars, and lots of food come roaring back into the eating pattern, under the pressure of family, entertainment, and dining out.

As previously noted, Toby's eating pattern illustrates each of the major eating problems of the overweight person. At the same time, it demonstrates that many people attempting to lose weight have enough technical information to do the job. Let's see how Toby, and you, can become healthy eaters.

Identifying High-Fat Foods

The first step in becoming a healthy eater is to be able to identify the high-fat foods in your diet consistently and regularly. Table 5.2 lists many of the common ones, correctly grouping them according to the food group in which they will be found: (1) bread, cereal, rice, and pasta; (2) vegetables; (3) fruits; (4) meat, poultry, fish, dry beans, eggs, and nuts; (5) milk, yogurt, and cheese. Although not a food group, the category of fats, oils, and sweets is also included in Table 5.2.

Although most of us know the common fatty foods, there are a few surprises here and there. So let's look at the food groups, qualitatively, for fat content.

• *Bread, cereal, rice, and pasta group.* This group might better have been named "Grains," because grain is the one valuable common component of foods within this group. Unfortunately, many grain-based foods contain ingredients that are not as valuable: Baked goods such as butter rolls, doughnuts, croissants, pancakes and waffles, high-fat or fried pastas, butter or cheese crackers, and granola are often filled with egg yolks, whole milk, and a spectrum of fats and oils.

• *Vegetable group.* This group generally contains healthful foods, but it also includes coconut, palm, and palm kernel oils, and the many foods made with these oils. Although these oils contain no cholesterol, they are highly saturated and contribute to raising cholesterol levels in the blood. Also certain foods in the vegetable group do contain healthier oils, but the oils are, of course, composed of fat and therefore just as calorie-intensive as the "bad" oils. Among these foods are olives, avocados, and peanuts. Corn and potatoes are valuable additions to any diet; however, when processed as corn chips or potato chips and deep-fried in whatever oil the manufacturer chooses to use, these vegetables lose their nutritional value.

• *Fruit group.* No fat!

• *Meat, poultry, fish, dry beans, eggs, and nuts group.* Among the prime grades of beef and other meats high in fat and cholesterol are hamburger; scrapple; spareribs; high-fat luncheon meats; canned, dried, and smoked meats; frankfurters and other sausages; and organ meats. Egg yolks, goose and duck (unless the fat is *very* well resolved), caviar, lox and Nova Scotia salmon, fish canned in oil, herring, and sardines are all high in fat.

• *Milk, yogurt, and cheese group.* In this group the fat is not at all hidden, as your taste buds will tell you. The worst offenders are milk products containing more than 1 percent fat, such as whole milk, condensed and evaporated milk; all kinds of creams, including sour cream; butter; nondairy cream substitutes made with coconut, palm, or palm kernel oils; ice cream; cream cheese; and most other cheeses. (Exception: Low-fat varieties of these products.)

TABLE 5.2 *Fat-Gram Content for Selected Fatty Foods*

LOW TO MEDIUM FAT
(Low Is Under 5 Grams per Serving;
Medium Is 5–10 Grams per Serving)

Breads, Cereals, Pasta, etc.	Low	Medium
Crackers, snack (4)		9.0
Cornbread from mix, 1 piece		5.8
Croissant, plain (½)	3.5	
Granola (1 oz.)		5.0
Muffin, blueberry, homemade (1 small)	3.7	
Muffin, bran, homemade (1 small)		5.1
Muffin, corn, homemade (1 small)	4.1	

Vegetables

	Low	Medium
Potatoes, French fried, frozen (10 strips)	4.4	
Potatoes, French fried, from restaurant (10 strips)		8.3
Potatoes, mashed (½ cup)	4.4	

Meat and Miscellaneous Foods

	Low	Medium
Bacon, broiled/pan-fried (3 slices)		9.4
Bologna, beef (1 slice)		6.6
Bologna, turkey (1 oz.)	4.7	
Burrito, bean (1)		5.0
Canadian bacon (2 slices)	3.9	
Chicken, fried, light meat w/o skin (3.5 oz.)		5.5
Chow mein (1 cup)		10.0
Egg, fried (1)		6.4
Egg, hard-boiled (1)		5.6
Egg, scrambled, w/milk and fat		7.1
Ham, 5% fat (1 slice)	1.4	
Hot dog, chicken		8.8
Lasagna, frozen, Banquet (4 oz.)		10.0
Pizza, cheese, homemade (1 slice)		8.6
Pork roast (3.5 oz.)		7.0
Roast beef, lean (3.5 oz.)		7.4
Salmon, canned, fish and bones (3 oz.)		5.1
Salmon, cooked by moist heat (3 oz.)		6.4

	Low	Medium
Sausage, fresh, cod link (2)		8.2
Soup, clam chowder, New England, canned (1 cup)		6.6
Soup, cream of tomato, Campbell's whole milk (1 cup)	2.2	
Tofu, raw (½ cup)	2.3	
Tuna, canned in oil, light (3 oz.)		7.0
Turkey, light and dark meat w/skin, roasted (3.5 oz.)		9.7

Milk, etc.

	Low	Medium
Cheese, American (1 oz.)		8.9
Cheese, brick (1 oz.)		8.4
Cheese, Cheddar (1 oz.)		9.4
Cheese, cottage, creamed (4 oz.)		5.1
Cheese, Monterey jack (1 oz.)		8.6
Cheese, mozzarella (1 oz.)		6.1
Cheese, mozzarella, part skim (1 oz.)	4.5	
Cheese, Muenster (1 oz.)		8.5
Cheese, Parmesan, grated (1 Tb.)	1.5	
Cheese, Swiss (1 oz.)		7.8
Ice milk, vanilla (1 cup)		5.6
Milk, chocolate, 1% (1 cup)	2.5	
Milk, chocolate, whole (1 cup)		8.5
Milk, 1% (1 cup)	2.6	
Milk, whole, 3.5% (1 cup)		8.0
Milk shake, thick, vanilla, large (1)		9.5
Pudding, instant (½ cup)	4.4	
Yogurt, plain, low fat (1 cup)	3.5	

Fats, Oils, and Sweets

	Low	Medium
Brownie, with nuts and chocolate icing	3.5	
Butter (1 tsp.)	4.1	
Chocolate chip cookies (2 small)	4.4	
Chocolate, milk, plain (1 oz.)		9.2
Corn chips (1 oz.)		8.8
Cream cheese (1 oz.)		9.9
Doughnut, cake type, plain (1)		5.8
Doughnut, glazed (1)		10.0
French dressing, regular (1 Tb.)		6.4

TABLE 5.2 *Fat-Gram Content for Selected Fatty Foods—continued*

	Low	Medium
Granola bar (1 bar)	4.2	
Italian dressing (1 Tb.)	1.5	
Margarine, stick, corn (1 tsp.)	3.8	
Oil and vinegar dressing, homemade (1 Tb.)		8.0
Popcorn, fat and salt added (1 cup)	2.0	
Sweet roll, cinnamon (1)	4.0	
Sweet roll, orange (1)		5.0
Tortilla chips, reg/nacho (1 oz.)		8.0

HIGH FAT
(10.1–15.0 Grams per Serving)

Vegetables

Potatoes, hash browns, homemade (½ cup)	10.9

Meat and Miscellaneous Foods

Burger King's Cheeseburger, regular (1)	15.0
Chicken, fried, light and dark meat (3 oz.)	13.6
Chili w/beans (1 cup)	14.0
Enchilada (12 oz.)	15.0
Fish sticks, frozen, batter-dipped, Van De Kamp's (4 oz.)	15.0
Ham, cured, regular, end (3.5 oz)	13.0
KFC's Original Recipe chicken breast, center (1)	13.7
Most nuts, mixed dry roasted (1 oz.)	14.6
Roast beef sandwich, on bun (1)	13.4
Roy Rogers roast beef sandwich (1)	10.1
Shrimp, breaded and fried (3 oz., 11 large)	10.4
Spaghetti with meat balls, canned or homemade (1 cup)	10.3
Steak, T-bone, broiled (3.5 oz.)	10.4
Submarine sandwich w/cold cuts and cheese (3″ to 4″)	11.0
Taco, Jack-in-the-Box, small (1)	11.0
Child's baked potato with cheese (1)	15.0
Child's chili serving	12.0

Milk, etc.

Ice cream, vanilla, rich, 16% fat (½ cup)	11.8
Ice cream, French vanilla, soft serve (½ cup)	11.2

Fats, Oils, and Sweets

Peanuts, dry roasted (1 oz.)	13.9
Peanuts, oil roasted (1 oz.)	14.0
Pie, apple homemade (⅛ pie)	11.9
Sunflower seeds, dry roasted (1 oz.)	14.1

HIGHER FAT
(15.1–20.0 Grams per Serving)

Vegetables

Avocado (½ medium)	15.0

Meat and Miscellaneous Foods

Chop suey (1 cup)	17.0
Dairy Queen's chili dog (1)	20.0
Enchilada, cheese (12 oz.)	19.0
Ground beef lean, broiled med. (3.5 oz.)	18.5
Hot dog, beef (1)	16.3
Italian sausage, pork, cod (1 link)	17.2
Macaroni and cheese, frozen, Banquet (1 cup)	17.0
McDonald's Egg McMuffin (1)	15.8
Peanut butter, creamy, smooth (2 Tb.)	16.4
Quiche, bacon and onion, pour-a-quiche (4.3 oz.)	18.0
Quiche Lorraine, frozen (7 oz.)	19.9
Steak, wedge-bone sirloin, broiled (3.5 oz.)	18.0
Top round, full cut, w/fat (3.5 oz.)	18.2
Tuna salad (½ cup)	19.0

Fats, Oils, and Sweets

Cheesecake (1 piece)	16.3
Sunflower seeds, oil roast (1 oz.)	16.3

TABLE 5.2 *Fat-Gram Content for Selected Fatty Foods—continued*

HIGHEST FAT
(20.1 Grams and Up per Serving)

Meat and Miscellaneous Foods

Arby's Roast Chicken Club (1)	33.0
Bratwurst, pork, cod (1 link)	22.0
Burger King's Double Cheeseburger w/bacon (1)	31.0
Burger King's Croissan'wich w/bacon, egg, and cheese (1)	24.0
Burger King's Ocean Catch fish fillet (1)	27.0
Burger King's Whaler (1)	27.0
Burger King's Whopper (1)	41.0
Chef's salad, ham and cheddar cheese (4.65 oz.)	28.1
Chicken pot pie, Banquet, frozen, baked (3 oz.)	24.0
Chicken pot pie, homemade (1 piece)	31.3
Ground beef, regular, medium broiled (3.5)	20.7
KFC's Extra Crispy chicken breast, center (1)	20.9
Macaroni and cheese, homemade (1 cup)	22.2
McDonald's Chicken McNuggets (1 serving)	21.3
McDonald's Filet O Fish (1)	25.7
McDonald's Big Mac (1)	35.0
McDonald's biscuit with sausage (1)	30.9
Pizza, Celeste (¼ of 19 oz. pie)	21.3
Pizza, Suprema, Celeste (9 oz. pie)	39.3
Pork chop, broiled, lean and fat sep. broiled (3.5 oz.)	22.1
Sausage, pork, smoked, link (1 link)	21.6
Spareribs lean and fat, braised (3.5 oz.)	30.3
Child's Big Classic	25.0

Fats, Oils, and Sweets

Pie, pecan, homemade (⅒ of 9″ pie)	23.6
Pizza Hut's supreme 10″ pizza (3 slices)	21.0

• *Fats, oils, and sweets group.* Foods in this category are grouped together for no logical reason other than to help you identify and avoid them. It is not necessary that you learn to identify what is contained in these foods, but you must know the other products in which these foods are hidden. Fats and oils are found in all fried foods; all solid fat, including butter, lard, and shortening; meat drippings and gravies; regular margarine; mayonnaise; conventionally baked pies, cookies (bakery and boxed), cakes (including cupcakes, fruitcakes, and snack cakes), and pastries; candy; nuts; various kinds of deep-fried chips; and cheese-based desserts. The word *sweets* refers to simple sugars, which are found wherever you see the word *sugar* on the ingredient list of packaged food. Ice cream is in a class by itself, containing the three most overused ingredients in the American diet—fat, sugar, and salt.

At this point, you may be asking yourself how you're going to manage the Take Control of Your Weight Program since everything you like seems to be included on the lists of foods to avoid.

Well, patience, patience. Let's work through your dietary analysis before making any dreary forecasts.

Analyzing Your Present Diet

Armed with the lists and descriptions provided herein, you are now ready to begin identifying the high-fat foods in your present diet. Remember that there are four other common problems in addition to high-fat eating: too much sugar and other simple carbohydrates, inconsistency of food choices over time, skipping meals with subsequent catching up, and eating the dreaded fourth meal. Following is a blank eating log to be used for recording your present eating pattern, and for designing your Take Control Eating Plan. (Please make as many photocopies of this page as you need, both for analyzing your present diet and eating patterns and for planning your new ones.)

First try to fill in from memory what you ate for each meal during the previous week. For most of us, this is not an easy task. After all, who remembers meals unless they are truly memorable, and these are often the ones we would most prefer to forget from a health standpoint anyway. However, trying your best to recall everything you have eaten over the past week will give you some idea of what you were eating before you began thinking about making some serious changes.

Next, without making any conscious changes in your eating, keep a log of

Eating Log

Day of Week	Breakfast	Lunch	Afternoon Snack	Dinner	Evening Snack
Mon. (Day 1)					
Tues. (Day 2)					
Wed. (Day 3)					
Thurs. (Day 4)					
Fri. (Day 5)					
Sat. (Day 6)					
Sun. (Day 7)					

what you eat this week. The two-week record should give you a fairly realistic picture of your diet and eating patterns. Now, using Table 5.2, the qualitative descriptions of high-fat foods, and your knowledge of the five common eating problems, list the high-fat foods and eating problems that appear on your log, and the frequency of both.

Having done that, you are ready to move on to the detailed planning of your Take Control of Your Weight Eating Plan. To do this you will have to know the available low-fat foods from which to choose.

Details of Healthy Eating

Low-Fat Eating

A simple list of some common nonfat and low-fat foods is presented in Table 5.3. However, you are not always going to carry around lists and tables with you. So, as we did with the high-fat foods, let's review the list of low-fat foods qualitatively.

• *Bread, cereal, rice, and pasta group.* All kinds of breads (so long as they are not covered with high-fat toppings; the more whole grain the flour, the less intrinsic fat the bread will have); pasta with low-fat sauces; oatmeal and other hot cereals; fortified cold cereals; whole-grain low-fat pancakes or waffles; low-fat matzoh, pita bread, and bread sticks (try whole wheat)

• *Vegetable group.* Salads (of course), stir-fried vegetables made with small amounts of vegetable oil, vegetable pizza, virtually any vegetable steamed or waterless cooked (topped with lemon juice, not butter)

• *Fruit group.* All fresh fruit, sherbet or sorbet, frozen fruit bars

• *Meat, poultry, fish, dry beans, eggs, and nuts group.* Lean red meat in small portions, skinned poultry, most fish, virtually all kinds of beans and peas, most shellfish (shrimp and lobster are low in fat but high in cholesterol)

• *Milk, yogurt, and cheese group.* 1% fat or skim milk, low- or nonfat yogurt, ice milk, low-fat or "lite" cheeses (check the labels), low-fat cottage cheese

• *Fats, oils, and sweets.* Gingersnaps, oatmeal cookies (check the label for fat content), fig bars, graham crackers (plain), pretzels (especially whole wheat for fiber), light or non-oil salad dressings (try lemon juice)

If you still don't find too much to entice you into making the change to low-fat eating, you will be interested in chapter 6, Healthy Shopping, Healthy Cooking. It introduces you to the wonderful world of tasty, appetizing, and attractive low-fat foods. Of course, you can't prepare and eat what you don't have at hand, so the chapter also shows you how to select the ingredients you need to build your menu of healthful dishes. You'll be surprised how much you

TABLE 5.3 *Selected Low-Fat Foods*

NONFAT

Breads, Cereals, Pasta, etc.
Corn flakes
Cream of wheat with skim milk
Macaroni, plain or vegetable
Rice, white
Rice, wild
Sugar frosted flakes

Vegetables
Broccoli
Cabbage
Carrot
Cauliflower
Celery
Corn
Green beans
Green peas
Green pepper
Greens
Lettuce
Pickle
Popcorn, air popped, unbuttered
Potato, baked
Snow peas
Spinach
Sweet potato, baked
Tomato, fresh
Tomato juice
Tossed salad, without dressing
Vegetable juice
Zucchini

Fruits
Apple
Applesauce
Cantaloupe
Fruit cocktail
Grapefruit
Grapes
Orange
Orange juice
Peaches
Pears
Pineapple
Prunes, dried, cooked
Prunes, dried, uncooked
Raisins
Strawberries
Watermelon

Meat, Dried Beans, etc.
Black-eyed peas, dried, cooked
Egg, hard-boiled, white only
Pinto beans, dried cooked

Milk, etc.
Milk, nonfat dry
Milk, skim
Yogurt, plain, nonfat

Fats, Oils, and Sweets
Angel food cake
Barbecue sauce
Catsup
Gelatin, flavored
Honey
Jelly
Maple syrup
Sugar

Beverages
Beer
Coffee
Soft drink, cola, low-calorie
Soft drink, cola, regular
Tea
Wine

LOWEST FAT
(1 Gram per Serving)

Breads, Cereals, Pasta, etc.
Bagel plain (½ bagel)
Bran flakes (1 oz.)
Bread, cracked wheat or whole
    wheat (1 slice)
Bread, pita (½)
Bread, pumpernickel or rye (1 slice)
Bread, white (1 slice)
Crackers, graham (2)
Crackers, rye (2)
Crackers, saltines (4)
Egg noodles, cooked
Hamburger bun (½)
Hard roll (½)
Hot dog bun (½)
Muffin, English, plain, toasted (½)
Oatmeal, instant, cooked
Raisin bran (1 oz.)
Rice, brown
Tortilla, corn (6")

Vegetables
Corn-on-the-cob, fresh, cooked (1
    ear)
Corn, canned, cream-style
Winter squash, fresh, baked (½ cup)

Fruits
Banana (1 medium)

Meat, Dried Beans, etc.
Baked beans (½ cup)
Black-eyed peas, canned (½ cup)
Flounder or sole, baked (3 oz.)
Navy beans (½ cup)
Refried beans, canned (½ cup)
Shrimp, boiled (3 oz.)
Soup, chicken noodle, dehydrated (1
    cup)

Milk, etc.
Cheese, cottage, 1% low-fat (½ cup)
Yogurt, frozen, plain (½ cup)

Fats, Oils, and Sweets
French dressing, low calorie (1 Tb.)
Gravy, beef, canned (¼ cup)
Mustard (1 Tb.)
Pretzels (1 oz.)

LOW FAT
(3 Grams per Serving)

Breads, Cereals, Pasta, etc.
Biscuit, from mix or refrigerated
    dough (1)
Crackers, whole wheat (2)
Dinner roll (1)
Pancake, plain or buckwheat (4")
Tortilla, flour (8")
Waffle, frozen (4")

Vegetables
Coleslaw (½ cup)
Popcorn, oil popped, unbuttered (1
    cup)
Sweet potato, candied (½ medium)

TABLE 5.3 *Selected Low-Fat Foods–continued*

Meat, Dried Beans, etc.	Milk, etc.
Chicken, roasted, without skin (3 oz.)	Buttermilk (1 cup)
	Cheese, cottage, 2% low-fat (½ cup)
Halibut, baked (3 oz.)	Cheese, Parmesan, grated (1 Tb.)
Soup, chicken noodle, canned (1 cup)	Coffee whitener, nondairy, liquid (1 Tb.)
Soup, Manhattan clam chowder with water (1 cup)	Half-and-half (1 Tb.)
	Ice milk (½ cup)
Soup, cream of tomato, with water (1 cup)	Light cream cheese (1 Tb.)
	Low-fat cheese (1 oz.)
Tuna, canned in water (3 oz.)	Milk, 1% low-fat (1 cup)
	Sour cream (1 Tb.)
	Yogurt, fruit flavored, low-fat (1 cup)

can enjoy low-fat eating, if you just take some time to learn how to shop and prepare the foods properly.

Low-Fat Food Choice Simplified

You have been presented with much information and a great deal of material to digest (please pardon the intended pun). You may be wondering if there are any *simple* ways to reduce fat in the diet. There certainly are and you probably know many of them already. But let's go over them once again.

• Substitute lower-fat for higher-fat milk, aiming toward 1% fat or skim milk. At first, many people think low-fat milk tastes strange, but after a while they think whole milk tastes too rich. Again, *gradual* is the byword. Go from whole milk to 2%, not to skim milk. The change will be painless. Next, go to 1% milk, and perhaps eventually to skim milk.

Yogurt is great, but to help you it must also be of the low-fat or nonfat variety. Plain, nonfat yogurt has many uses, from becoming a substitute for butter, margarine, or sour cream on baked potatoes, to being the base for a vegetable spread.

• Eat red meat sparingly, though you do not have to eliminate it completely. Gradually begin sampling the cuts lower in fat until you find a few you'd be happy to add to your menu. Low-fat cuts of beef are flank steak, eye of round, top round, sirloin, tenderloin; low-fat pork is center-cut loin chops; lamb is loin chops and leg of lamb. With all meat and poultry, be sure to trim any visible fat, and eat only a portion of about 3 ounces.

Extra lean and lean hamburger still provide about 60 percent of their calories from fat.

• Sausages, hot dogs, and luncheon meats should almost always be avoided. The sooner you wean yourself from these meat products the better. Even poultry luncheon meats and hot dogs are not all low in fat, though they are often lower in cholesterol than those made with red meats. Interestingly enough, some luncheon meats, such as boiled ham, are low in fat. (Chapter 6 teaches you how to read labels.)

• Carbohydrates are super foods and can be prepared very tastily (see chapter 6). As you develop your low-fat eating habits, you will increasingly find yourself focusing your eating on low-fat, high-carbohydrate foods: beans (contrary to past belief, beans are definitely not fattening), rice, potatoes, pasta, whole-grain cereals, bread and bread products (such as bagels), green and orange vegetables, and fruit. (Even the "starch" subgroup of the carbohydrates is healthful, as long as it's not loaded down with fatty toppings.)

We've all heard the apparently incongruous advice that you can eat as much as you want of carbohydrates and still lose weight. The trick is that carbohydrates give you a "full" feeling sooner than do fats and proteins; therefore, you tend to eat less even while you may be eating as much as you want. Remember, however, that you can lose much of the dietary advantages of carbohydrates if you cover them with high-fat toppings.

• Not all chicken is the same. Choose white meat, and remove the skin. Unlike cows and pigs, chickens and turkeys carry most of their fat under the skin, not as marbling in and around muscles (although in the dark meat of poultry there is some fat too). Beware of ground turkey and chicken; they are usually high in fat, probably because much more dark than white meat is used. As well, on occasion, skin and fat from other parts of the bird are also included. It's a good idea to look for the label "lean" on your ground turkey.

• Try serving salad dressing, even the light or no-oil varieties, on the side, rather than putting the dressing over the entire salad. Dip each forkful of salad into the dressing; you will find that you eat less dressing.

• Substitute frozen low- or nonfat yogurt, ice milk, or sherbet, for ice cream; then move to fruit sorbets and frozen fruit bars.

• The lower-fat varieties of fish include cod, haddock, northern pike, flounder, grouper, halibut, red snapper, Dover sole, bass, bluefish, shark (technically not a fish, by the way), swordfish, and tuna. Higher-fat varieties are coho salmon, mackerel, pompano, and sardines. Beware of tuna packed in oil (usually vegetable, not fish oil) and tuna salad made with mayonnaise.

• For quick and easy dinner preparation, don't be afraid to try frozen light meals, though you must always read the labels to make sure they really are low in fat.

• Beware of butter. It tastes great, but it is 100 percent fat (as is regular margarine). Use low-fat margarine instead of butter. If you read the label, you may be surprised at the fat content in margarine, even in those described as low-fat. Use lemon juice instead of margarine, especially as a topping for vegetables. If you gradually reduce the amount of whatever spread you use on bread, crackers, matzoh, etc., you'll find that you quickly become accustomed to the reduction. It's a different taste, but an easy one to get used to.

• Make sure to skim the fat from homemade soup.

• Use pureed fruit instead of whipped toppings. Instead of jellies and jams, purchase fruit preserves made solely of fruit with no added sugar. You can use them as toppings on hot cereal as well as on many other dishes that need something to improve appearance and taste. If you must use mayonnaise, use the light variety.

Dealing with Refined Sugar

Fruits and vegetables contain both simple and complex carbohydrates (the terms *simple* and *complex* refer to the chemical structure of their molecules). Simple carbohydrates include foodstuffs such as refined (table) sugar and the alcohol in alcoholic beverages. Simple carbohydrates contain no fat but carry "empty calories"—that is, unlike the complex carbohydrates, the simple ones have neither nutrients like vitamins and minerals, nor fiber.

Contrary to popular belief, small quantities of simple carbohydrates are not the real villains in the weight-gain process. For example, one teaspoon of refined sugar contains only 18 calories. Alcoholic beverages, however, contain enormous quantities of calories (the term "beer belly" is not a misnomer). But the primary weight-control problem created by sweet foods—cookies, candy, cakes, pies, ice cream, and so forth—is not the refined sugar content but rather the fat content. Because fats also provide tenderness, moisture, and flavor, virtually all sweet foods are brimming with fat. It is the combination of sugar and fat that makes rich desserts taste so good.

If you have low-calorie overweight (LCO), you probably do not eat very many sweets. But if you have normal or high-calorie overweight, or if you are dealing with LCO and are successfully raising your resting metabolic rate, you need to be concerned with overall caloric intake. A low-fat label does not guarantee that the food is low in calories. Eight ounces of Entenmann's nonfat cakes contain 560 calories. Occasionally eating some low-fat high-calorie foods will not hurt you, but if they are currently staples in your diet you should start easing them out. You certainly don't want to replace the fat in your diet with refined sugar.

Devising Your TCYW Eating Plan

Okay. You are taking control, assuming responsibility. You don't need gimmicks any longer; you know they don't work. You understand that it is only gradual change in eating and exercise that can lead you to success in the long run.

The initial phase of the Take Control of Your Weight Eating Plan is 28 days. Since it is *your* diet, the first step you are going to take is to plan it.

Most diets ask you to begin without any specific preparation. The Take Control Eating Plan is different. Even the starting day is your decision. In many diets Day 1 is always a Monday. In this program you choose Day 1, a Take Control Do-It Day on which to start. Monday may be good, but Saturday or Thursday may be better for you. So the Take Control of Your Weight Eating Plan begins on *your* Day 1. The keys, of course, are gradual change and food substitution. Let's review those principles briefly.

Food Substitution and Gradual Change

You have been shown why calorie counting and menu plans do not and cannot work for many people. Food substitution is much easier, much more satisfying, and much more effective. The goal is to achieve *qualitative* change in your eating. Counting fat grams and budgeting your food fat are certainly ways to do that, but most people will not continue that method for very long.

If you reduce high-fat foods and increase low-fat foods, you will achieve your goal without actually having to count fat grams or calories. And you will achieve permanent change if you engage in food substitution gradually. Gradual change means just that. You won't be trying to do everything at once, become discouraged, and in the end accomplish nothing. You will put into place a series of small changes. Remember, one success per week adds up to 52 successes in one year.

Do you eat four meals a day, every day? Well, in the first week of your Take Control Eating Plan, you can cut out or convert to fruit one of those seven midnight snacks. Then the next week convert two of them. Drop another one in the third week, and so forth. Do you never eat breakfast during the week? Well, in your first week try to have breakfast once, let us say on Wednesday. The following week you can have a Monday breakfast. Before you know it, you will be eating breakfast every day.

You do not have to stop eating chocolate, ice cream, red meat, cheese, and butter from Day 1. You have time and power to bring about the changes. Do you now eat red meat five times a week? Well, how about cutting it to four times for the first two weeks of the Take Control Eating Plan and if that goes well, how about to three times for the next two weeks? Do you believe that in the end you really won't be able to do without red meat at least twice a week? Fine. Set that number as your goal, and as you gradually reduce the frequency, consider substituting low-fat varieties of red meat for the high-fat cuts you now eat.

In the planning phase, you will go through this process for all the major foods you have identified as being problems and contributing to your overweight. You will also decide what foods you want to substitute. You may have found all these new food items a bit off-putting as you worked your way through the lists. But recall there is information later in this book that will show you how you can make low-fat eating very tasty, if you invest some time and effort.

But before we get to that, let's prepare your Take Control Eating Plan.

Begin to Change—Gradually

Make four copies of the blank eating log (page 80), one for each of the four weeks of the eating plan. Analyze your present eating log to identify all of your eating problems. (Toby, you may remember, happens to have all five; not every reader will.) In putting together and implementing your eating plan, tackle each of the eating problems you have during a separate week. Each week, you will maintain and enhance the new behaviors developed as further changes are made.

Suppose that you decide to deal with high-fat eating first. Using the high-fat food lists, you may identify whole milk, cream, cheese, butter, fried foods, red meat, baked goods, and candy as problems. In the first week, you will begin to reduce dietary fat, making substitutions of low- or lower-fat products for some of those with the most fat. You will not try to eliminate all high-fat foods at once, but will choose the correct pace at which to proceed and which foods will be the first to be eliminated.

If you are like Toby, who ate red meat seven times in the sample week, your first step in dealing with this problem is to set a long-term objective for frequency, perhaps eating red meat only twice a week. Will you go from seven to two in that first week? That's part of the prescription for failure followed by many weight-loss plans. A better first step is to cut the frequency to six times, perhaps to five. Thus, if the frequency of eating red meat is reduced by just one meal over each of the first four weeks of the Take Control of Your Weight Eating Plan, at the end of a month you will almost have reached your goal. And you will not have the stress of dealing with a too-sudden change in diet.

At the same time, you will be substituting healthy, tasty foods for the red meat, selecting from Table 5.3 (pages 82–84) and the additional qualitative lists. You can also look to previous experience to help the process. For example, chicken, fish, and vegetarian meals may have been included once or twice during your sample eating week. It is simply a matter of slowly increasing the frequency of those kinds of meals. This book will advise you and help you analyze and make decisions for each of the dietary high-fat foods identified.

In the second week, you will add another piece of the puzzle, perhaps inconsistency in food choices. Inconsistency is harmful because it tricks you into thinking that you are doing something useful for weight loss when you are not, and because it entices you to go back to your old ways. On Toby's Eating Log, for example, Toby's main course for dinner on Monday was healthy, but he added chocolate fudge cake for dessert; then he attempted to balance potato chips with a diet soda. Friday's eating pattern, healthy the whole day, is completely inconsistent with the rest of the week. Toby will learn that Friday's isolated healthy eating pattern will contribute little to a permanent change in eating habits. At the same time, Toby should feel encouraged because he has the underlying knowledge of what healthy eating should be.

Although the Take Control of Your Weight Eating Plan will help you permanently change your eating patterns, don't think that you can *never* have a piece of chocolate fudge cake, mud pie, or pie à la mode. Of course you can, and will. Remember, perfectionism is *not* on the menu of this program. However, when you are starting your new eating plan, it will help for the first few weeks to establish a consistent pattern of healthy eating. Also, you want to make sure that when you do have that marshmallow sundae, you do it by choice, under control.

The gradual-change process will continue, again using Tables 5.2 and 5.3. For example, you may decide to add cream to your coffee only every other time, to eat homemade popcorn with only half your usual amount of butter, or better yet a vegetable spray, and to have plain unbuttered popcorn at the movies.

(Some movie theaters now offer unsalted, unbuttered popcorn. Ask for it!) On the other hand, you will realize that using a light salad dressing as part of an otherwise high-fat meal is just kidding yourself.

Since the Take Control of Your Weight Eating Plan works through learned behavior, and from the beginning uses healthy eating as the way to lose weight, there is no artificial, discrete maintenance phase. From the beginning you will know that the only way to keep off lost weight is to make permanent, healthy changes in eating. You will see phase one of the Take Control Eating Plan as the first four weeks of the rest of your life and will concentrate on establishing an eating change continuum. You will also know that you will not be able to, nor should you, achieve all of your goals for eating, weight loss, and exercise during the first four weeks. However, once the pattern of gradual change is established, it can continue indefinitely, leading to progressive opening of new vistas and self-improvement.

Tasty Low-Fat Food Preparations
and Healthy Meals

It's one thing to identify foods that are healthy, quite another to make tasty, nutritious meals from them. Unless you are one of those relatively rare people who can eat the same foods over and over again, you are not going to stay with healthy eating unless your meals look good, smell good, and taste good. Also, your family members want to enjoy meals with you, even if they don't have weight problems themselves. What can you do? Find or create meals that are healthy, using foods that look good, taste good, and are good for you.

There are many low-fat cookbooks on the market that contain plenty of recipes—ranging from simple to complex—for healthy, low-fat dishes that are both delicious and satisfying. Chapter 6 presents guides to some of the good-tasting healthy eating available to you. In the meantime, let's discuss some of the simple ways you can cut fat from your diet without searching through cookbooks, recipes, and menu planners.

Simple Healthy Eating
Daily Meals

The old maxim "eat three square meals a day" is very valid. Many people think that skipping breakfast, and the calories and fat it might contain, is a good way to lose weight. Experience shows that this is not the case. In fact, studies show that regularity of eating is an element of successful weight loss that can be as important as the content of the meals.

People who begin the day with a balanced breakfast and eat regular meals during the day, tend to manage their weight better than those who don't eat breakfast. One reason is that people who skip breakfast tend to eat more later in the day, especially the dreaded fourth meal (which becomes the third meal, often eaten as a high-fat midnight snack). Furthermore, the long period from last night's dinner to today's lunch will leave you without energy. Your compensation for this may be a late-morning coffee and doughnut whose calories you may not bother to count but which can include more fat and simple sugar than a wholesome, full breakfast. Having breakfast will also give you more energy in the morning, helping you to function optimally until lunchtime.

Skipping lunch will tempt you into destructive snacks in the late afternoon. In addition, skipping meals, either breakfast or lunch, will probably cause you to eat too much at the next meal. Therefore, *not* skipping meals and *not* eating the fourth meal or other unhealthy snacks are both equally important elements in the Take Control of Your Weight Eating Plan.

Breakfast *is* easy to skip. You think you're doing something positive for your weight and you're in a hurry anyway. Breakfast is also an easy meal to fill with fat. So, what can you do? The most important thing is to be prepared. Keep in mind those breakfast food choices that are tasty, filling, and healthy all at the same time. Chapter 6 presents a detailed discussion of breakfast foods, but here are some that require little preparation:

• Nonfat or low-fat hot cereals such as oatmeal are excellent, but for many of us the flavor needs to be improved. Most cereals are healthy and come from the food group from which we should choose 6 to 12 servings a day. Oatmeal provides the additional benefit of oat bran, which can help reduce cholesterol levels in some people.

Again we see the insidious hand of habit: Many of us learned in childhood to sprinkle table sugar on hot cereal. When people lived more active lives, sugar on hot cereal was not a problem, because a long day of hard manual labor was the norm. For active children, sugar on hot cereal still may not be a problem, except for the danger of dental caries. But some of us rejected hot cereal when we learned that refined sugar is bad for us, because the two seemed to go together like bread and butter; thus, we eliminated a very healthy food from our diets.

Pure fruit preserves is an excellent choice of topping for hot cereal. You can also mix in some raisins while the cereal is cooking. And, you can use cold fresh fruit on both hot and cold cereal. But if you will eat hot cereal only with sugar, go ahead and do so. Remember, sugar provides only 18 calories per teaspoon. You can also use honey (although honey has more calories than sugar—65 compared to 54 per tablespoon) and canned fruit. Once you are in the habit of eating hot cereal, you might gradually eliminate the sugar or honey, substituting unsweetened fruit or fruit preserves one or two mornings a week and, gradually, every morning.

We don't always have the need to sweeten cold cereal, because alas, in many cases the manufacturer has done it for us. When shopping for cold cereals, be careful to read labels (see chapter 6), not only to find the sugar but also to help choose low-fat varieties. High fiber is a desirable extra.

Be sure to use low- or nonfat milk. Also you can try moistening cold cereal with fruit juice. Some people really like it that way.

• Breads such as bagels and English muffins and bran, corn, and fruit muffins are all good choices, so long as they don't have high-fat contents and you don't smear them with high-fat spreads. You can tell if a muffin is fatty by rubbing it on a paper napkin; greasy muffins leave a transparent stain. You can also tell by lifting it; if the muffin feels too heavy for its size, you can be sure that it was made with a lot of fat. Do you like waffles or pancakes? See the cooking section in Suggested Readings and General References for a list of cookbooks that contain tempting recipes. As a rule, whole-grain breads are preferable.

• Fruit jam in modest quantities is a fine spread that contains carbohydrate calories but little or no fat. Try it on any bread without first applying a fat-based spread.

• Still like eggs? Well, if you're eating them four or five times per week, cut back gradually, just as you will be doing with other high-cholesterol foods. (The American Heart Association says 2 or 3 egg yolks a week is okay.) You can use low- or nonfat egg substitutes to make scrambled eggs and omelettes. See chapter 6 for some specifics on eggs.

• Low- or nonfat yogurt can be used in many ways, such as a topping on cereal and fruit or as the base with fruit and/or low-fat granola added.

Is it best not to snack? By and large, yes. If you get hungry between meals, your body will be forced to draw on your fat stores for energy. But, if you get too hungry, the likelihood is that when you eat your next meal you will eat more than you really need to satisfy your body's energy requirements. And many of us *like* to snack, whether between meals or before bedtime. The secret, especially at bedtime, is to avoid transforming a quick, light, healthful snack into a fourth meal.

Here are some healthy substitutes for common high-fat snack foods:

• Fruit is the best snack, of course. But if you're used to eating cheese, potato chips, and candy bars for snacks, you will need time to adjust to the changeover. Make the change gradually, dropping one snack each week. Choose fresh fruits in season. Pure fruit juices are great too, but avoid "fruit drinks," which add corn syrup or other sweeteners. Dried fruit is fine from time to time, but only in moderation. Dried fruit has no fat but is generally so condensed that it is high in calories per unit of weight (over 400 in one cup of raisins). Sherbet, lower-calorie sorbet, and frozen fruit sticks are good choices.

• Whole wheat low-fat crackers and bread sticks and low-fat cookies and pretzels are especially good choices. Yes, you did see cookies in the listing. Look for gingersnaps, fig bars, and fruit cookies, but you must read labels (see chapter 6). You must also be careful not to overindulge: Low-fat food can quickly become high-fat if you eat a lot of it. Don't forget graham crackers with cinnamon for a tasty and crunchy treat. Note that palm and coconut oils have been popular ingredients in commercially prepared cookies; both are high in saturated fat. Although most American food manufacturers have stopped using these oils in baked goods, you should continue checking labels for them.

• Vegetables such as raw carrot sticks and celery are the classic dieter's rabbit food. They are good and good for you, but can certainly be uninteresting. Try making up one of the low- or nonfat yogurt dips you can find in many low-fat cookbooks. Also, think about eating plain green or red peppers (plenty of taste on their own) and radishes (the good ones have plenty of snap). Air-popped popcorn is great stuff and tends to be filling, but goes from a plus to a minus if you add butter (try a light coating of vegetable spray instead). Dry cereals containing fruits and nuts make a great snack, dry, right out of the box. But you must be careful when buying such snacks. For example, some commercial granola is loaded with fat. Check the label.

• Nonfat or low-fat yogurt should become a staple in your refrigerator because it has so many healthy uses, including breakfast food, veggie dips, and topping for a baked potato that you have as a snack or as part of dinner. If you must have cheese, try modest amounts of the low-fat varieties.

Eating in Restaurants

Eating out and eating healthy can sound like a contradiction in terms. But you can do both with some advance planning.

The most important element is choosing the restaurant. Many restaurants offer low-fat items on their menus, but you will have difficulty finding them in chicken-and-rib or roast-beef-and-steak houses. However, even in those restaurants you should be able to find dishes relatively low in fat. Order chicken (remove the skin if it's still on), seafood (*not* in cream or cheese sauces), or fish (broiled, not fried; and plain, not coated with batter or butter).

The following kinds of restaurants offer the best opportunities for low-fat eating: Italian (choose pasta with low-fat toppings such as marsala, marinara, and primavera; avoid cheese, unless it's a low-fat one such as Parmagiano Reggiano); Chinese (have stir-fried or steamed dishes); Japanese (stay away from tempura); Mexican (have lots of rice and beans; avoid sour cream, shredded cheese, and guacamole); Indian (already light on the meat, heavy on rice, vegetables, and breads); French (make sure the cooking is Provençale, which is based on olive oil, not cream sauce). In any restaurant, ask about any low-fat dishes they may have.

If the menu has an American Heart Association "Heart Healthy" or other low-fat eating section, try it. You may be surprised by how tasty some of the selections are.

If you are hungry when you arrive at the restaurant, don't dive into the fat-fried chips, such as crisp Chinese noodles or tortillas, which are often provided before you order your meal. Don't eat three slices of bread covered with thick slabs of butter before you order your meal. Try bread with no butter or just a thin coating, bread sticks (plain), or the crudités (raw veggies) that some restaurants provide. If you order a dinner that includes the salad bar, make up your own plate of crudités before you assemble your dinner salad.

"Belly up to the salad bar," as one of my colleagues, the nutritionist Virginia Aronson, is fond of saying. As you know, complex carbohydrates will fill you up fast. If the restaurant offers the salad bar as a main-course option, you might find that a soup (try gazpacho, a spicy, Spanish-style, tomato-based soup) or seafood appetizer combined with the as-much-as-you-can-eat salad will work fine for you. Emphasize fresh vegetables and beans. If bread is offered and there is a whole-grain variety, select that one for the fiber content. Stay away from coleslaw and chicken, potato, and macaroni salads, all usually made with mayonnaise.

Most salad dressings provided at salad bars are high in fat. A couple of ladles of the stuff can ruin the most carefully chosen salad. So, choose one of the low-fat or light dressings. If none is offered, use oil and vinegar, or lemon juice, with fresh pepper. Unless the dressing is entirely nonfat take it on the side in a cup or small bowl, and dip your forkfuls of salad into it. Avoid toppings such as cheese, bacon bits, and deep-fried croutons. Use the seeds and raisins.

Dessert? If you have eaten a low-fat dinner, and you have a craving for a really rich dessert, go ahead and indulge that craving. But do not eat an entire serving. Ask a fellow diner or two to share that piece of cheesecake with you. Often you will find that a bite or three is all you need to satisfy your craving. You may not find it difficult to forgo the rich chocolate desserts that many restaurants emphasize, because many low-fat eaters rapidly develop a low tolerance for chocolate. Have the strawberries with a touch of whipped cream or the melon with a scoop of sherbet. A good compromise is fruit pie—not à la mode, of course.

Eating Fast Food

Healthy eating in fast-food restaurants offers special challenges, but it can be done. Awareness is the first skill you must develop. You may know that the triple-decker cheeseburger is loaded with fat, and that adding only one thin slice of processed American cheese to a simple hamburger increases its fat content significantly. But did you know that one serving of processed chicken chunks or one deep-fried, coated fish filet sandwich actually has more fat than a quarter-pound hamburger? Or that a grilled chicken sandwich can be made into a fat nightmare by the addition of the restaurant's special sauce? And that deep-fried chicken, with the skin, may offer as much fat as the gooeyest hamburger special?

So, you have to be careful, but you certainly do not have to risk armed rebellion among your children by completely avoiding fast-food places forever. Want a hamburger? Have it prepared plain, no cheese, no sauce, no bacon. Want toppings? Choose lettuce, tomato, onion. Roast beef sandwiches and beef (or chicken) fajitas usually contain less fat than a hamburger. And there are lean hamburgers, which still taste good.

Chicken is a great choice, but choose a grilled chicken sandwich without the special sauce. If you must have deep-fried chicken pieces, remove the coating and skin, and hold each piece up for a few seconds to let the fat drip out. It will still taste good (although after doing that a few times, you may never order that particular meal again). The same advice generally applies to fish.

Baked potatoes? Of course, but avoid the cheese and bacon dressings. Ask for chives and low-fat sour cream. If they don't have it, ask if you can add your own toppings, from the salad or toppings bar. Pizza is relatively healthy, especially if you do not order extra cheese and stick to the vegetable toppings (peppers, onions, and mushrooms) rather than the pepperoni or sausage. Mexican fast-food establishments can provide you with low-fat alternatives, as long as you choose soft rather than crisp (deep-fried) tacos; order the veggies, beans, and chicken; and avoid beef, cheese toppings, sour cream, and guacamole.

Salads? Yes, naturally. If the salad is a packaged one, be sure to stay away from the chef's salad (usually loaded with fatty meat and cheese) and select a low-fat dressing.

Don't ignore the local deli. You can find a wide variety of low-fat salads, hot and cold pastas, and low-fat sandwiches made with (fresh, not processed) turkey, chicken, and other low-fat meats and cheese.

Vitamin Supplements

Vitamin supplements are a multibillion-dollar industry in our country. They are also the focus of a rather heated debate. While everyone agrees that vitamins are absolutely essential to the maintenance of our health and well-being, opinions differ about the need to take supplements.

Some people maintain that if you eat a balanced diet you will receive enough vitamins and other nutrients such as minerals.

Others maintain that few of us eat a sufficiently balanced diet. They add that nutrients are reduced substantially during growth, storage, transport, processing, and preparation of the foods we eat; therefore, we could not possibly obtain the proper amount of vitamins and minerals. So, we should take supplements.

A third group argues that certain naturally available vitamins, if taken in large doses not ordinarily available in even the purest of foods, can diminish the risk of certain cancers and other diseases.

The balanced-diet group contend that many of the dollars we spend on vitamins and other food supplements are literally flushed down the toilet. Most people's bodies cannot use amounts of vitamins and minerals in excess of the Recommended Dietary Allowances (RDAs) established by the National Academy of Sciences. According to this view, for most people the RDAs (which vary by age and sex) are satisfied by eating a balanced diet. Furthermore, if you take a supplement, only some of it is excreted. The body cannot eliminate superfluous amounts of certain vitamins, which are then stored. If accumulation of vitamins such as A and D becomes excessive, the effect can be toxic.

There is strong disagreement about whether or not the foods we buy are vitamin depleted. However, it is well established that vitamins will not provide extra energy, as implied by some vitamin advertising. Nor will iron wake you up. You need to take an iron supplement only if you have been diagnosed as having iron-deficiency anemia (low iron in the blood). But if your blood iron level is normal, taking additional iron will not wake you up and may actually harm you. Energy comes from calories, not from vitamins.

In recent years several scientific studies have been published that provide increasing evidence that vitamins A (in the form of beta carotene), folic acid (a B vitamin), C, D, E, K, niacin, and the mineral selenium, when taken in sufficient amounts, may reduce the risk for certain diseases.

In any case, eat plenty of the foods that provide vitamins and minerals naturally. Fruits, vegetables, and grains abound in those nutrients. When deciding on taking supplements for other purposes, proceed with caution. If you have been diagnosed by a registered dietician or physician as having a special need for a specific vitamin or mineral, you should take that specific vitamin or mineral supplement(s) as prescribed. There is no evidence to date that consuming large amounts of vitamin and mineral supplements in an indiscriminate fashion has any beneficial effects whatsoever.

Behavioral Interventions

If you have previously tried to lose weight, whether on your own or in an organized program, you are probably familiar with the term *behavioral modification,* or "behavior mod" for short. And most likely you have been introduced to its components. Behavioral modification is a psychological intervention designed to change behavior directly, without addressing intermediate mental processes. Its basic assumption is that changes in behavior can precede changes in thinking and feeling, and, in fact, can be instrumental in causing changes in thinking and feeling.

With behavioral modification, you consciously take control of a behavior, focusing on outcome rather than on the psychological and metabolic genesis of the activities you are trying to change. In essence, behavioral modification is a combination of the "Just Do It" and "Just Say No" approaches. Used correctly in the ideal situation by the right candidate, it can and does work. However, by itself it is *not* a way to lose weight, directly. Weight loss is only achieved by the combination of calorie restriction, activity increase, *and* alteration of the metabolism that is right for you. Behavioral modification is an intervention that can help you to restrict calorie intake, increase activity, and thereby modify your metabolism, but it will not necessarily lead to a loss in weight. It will do so only if the behavioral changes achieved produce changes in *your* eating patterns that can actually lead to weight loss for *you*. And that, of course, depends very much on what kind of overweight you have in the first place.

If you have low-calorie overweight, and you use these techniques simply to reduce your calorie intake further, you will not only fail to lose weight, but may also harm your metabolism more, contributing to eventual weight gain. On the other hand, certain behavioral techniques can be very helpful in lowering the *fat* in your diet. So, you have to be careful in applying behavioral modification techniques, to make sure that if they do succeed in and of themselves they truly will be helping you to achieve the ultimate goals you have set for yourself. In sum, behavioral modification can be used to help you eat less generally or less fat specifically. But again, it will not automatically lead to weight loss and is, therefore, not a panacea.

The following behavioral modification techniques can help you eat less or eat less fat:

- Keep an eating log to help you focus on your particular eating problems.
- Control mindless eating (eating for reasons other than to satisfy hunger), and increase awareness of unconscious dietary habits such as nibbling foods that add fat to your diet.
- Eat only three meals a day, consciously avoiding the fourth meal.
- Eat only when you're hungry. Learn the cues that compel you to eat when you are not hungry and learn how to handle them; identify the nonhunger triggers that cause you to eat.
- Stop eating once you feel full.
- Do nothing else when you eat.
- Sit down to eat, and stay there until you're finished.
- Eat slowly (take smaller bites, chew completely, do not fill your mouth with food, put only one kind of food in your mouth at a time, place your fork on your plate between bites).
- Reduce portion size, reject second helpings, and consciously avoid the habit of necessarily eating everything on your plate.
- Control snacking.

• Develop smart shopping habits (see Chapter 6): Plan your shopping trips carefully; use a list; shop on a full stomach, so as not to be tempted into making high-fat impulse purchases.

• Do not buy high-fat foods, or, if you do, keep them out of sight at home.

• Do not feel shy or wasteful about throwing out high-fat foods that you purchased by mistake, brought home in a doggie bag, or received as a gift.

6

Healthy Shopping, Healthy Cooking

Low-Fat Eating Begins in the Supermarket

You have read chapter 5, identified the high-fat components of your diet, and made a list of food substitutes you are going to gradually introduce into your diet. Now you are ready to begin the process of implementing your Take Control of Your Weight Eating Plan. But, you don't start at your dining-room table; your first steps will be taken in your supermarket, farmers market, or local grocery store.

Shopping for food is where it all begins, where you start to take control of your eating. If you don't have unhealthy food in the house, you can't eat it. If you have low- and nonfat foods in the house, you will eat them.

Planning

Planning is a critical element in this whole process. Every endeavor needs a plan if it is to have the desired outcome. It is a critical element for achieving success in most endeavors, from creating economic security for retirement to successful coaching in sports.

Meal planning is essentially the process of preselecting foods that meet two criteria: they should satisfy your calorie/fat needs, and you should like them. By planning, you make sure that decisions about which foods to eat are not made on the basis of what happens to be on hand. Common sense and experience prove that if you don't plan that trade of high-fat cheese and crackers for an orange and low-fat granola, it will not take place. In eating, as in many other activities, spontaneity is the handmaiden of habit. Therefore, if you want to change eating habits, meal planning becomes an essential and powerful tool for success.

Preparing for the Supermarket

If you have completed your dietary analysis and written your substitutes list, you are prepared for the next step. If you intend to eat gourmet low-fat meals, you should choose 30 to 40 recipes in advance. Review them and list the common ingredients. Then make sure you have all of those stock ingredients in the house, so that you won't become frustrated by lack of important ingredients when you are ready to prepare the recipes. This frustration can cause you to abandon a low-fat recipe and put a hamburger in a frypan instead.

Making lists is essential because you want to purchase only the foodstuffs you need. In addition, you may be shopping in new sections of the market and cannot rely on memory as you shop. Become familiar with the sections of the market you use regularly, especially the sections where low-fat foodstuffs are shelved. For example, some supermarkets stock low- and nonfat salad dressings with other low-fat foods, while others stock them with regular salad dressings.

Stick to your list. Don't subject yourself to excessive temptation by browsing through impulse items, often high in fat and placed strategically on the shelves to lure the undisciplined shopper. Avoid impulse buying and purchasing foods on sale simply because they are on sale. Often they are high-fat items. At the same time, be aware of special sales on low-fat items.

By the way, if you currently eat substantial amounts of red meat, you may save money by reducing the red meat in your diet and eating low-fat foods. The foods you will substitute for red meat generally cost less. Although you will be eating more chicken and fish (fish may not be cheaper per pound than red meat), you will probably eat smaller portions than the red meat portions you ate previously.

Never shop when you are hungry. Hungry shoppers tend to buy more food and more high-fat food than shoppers who are not hungry. They are also more vulnerable to impulse buying.

The One-Week Eating Plan

One of the best ways to shop healthy is to prepare your list from a one-week eating plan. On the following pages, you will find a one-week plan that Toby, our Take Control planner from chapter 5, might construct two or three months into the program. Comparing this plan to Toby's original eating log (see pages 70–71) you can see that Toby has made some substitutions and is gradually changing. Toby's new plan presents a healthier eating pattern developed from his original pattern. The model is intended to illustrate how gradual change and food substitution can be accomplished, in a rather painless way when given time and attention. We are not suggesting that you follow Toby's plan; it does not apply to everyone indiscriminately. For your plan to be effective, develop what will be appropriate for your Pathway Down and appropriate for your eating pattern, your needs, your predilections, your rate of change—what works best for you.

Toby on the Road to Healthy Eating

Day of Week	Breakfast	Lunch	Afternoon Snack	Dinner	Evening Snack
Mon.	Low-fat cereal w/ 1% milk & banana Eng. muffin w/low-fat marg. Coffee, w/ low-fat creamer	Broiled chicken sand. w/let. & tom. Baked pot. w/low-fat topping Diet soda	Coffee w/ low-fat creamer Two low-fat cookies	Mustard-baked chicken w/ rice Lemon broccoli Red cabbage and bean sprouts w/ low-fat dressing Angel food cake	Low-fat granola Diet soda
Tues.	Oat cereal w/1% milk 7-grain toast w/ low-fat marg. and jam Fruit juice	Oriental chicken salad w/ low-fat dressing Low-fat crackers Diet soda	None	Meatloaf made w/ lean ground beef Oven fries Grilled herb tomatoes Green salad w/light dressing Fruit sorbet	Fresh fruit Graham crackers

Day of Week	Breakfast	Lunch	Afternoon Snack	Dinner	Evening Snack
Wed.	Same as Monday, but a different cereal	Pita bread w/ tabbouleh Fresh fruit Fruit juice	Four fig bars Coffee w/ low-fat creamer	Broiled fish, Cajun style Cajun rice Grilled string beans w/garlic Gelatin w/ low-fat topping	None
Thurs.	Scrambled eggs w/ Can. bacon Toasted bagel w/ low-fat marg. Fruit juice Coffee w/ low-fat creamer	Low-fat yogurt w/ fresh fruit Oat bran muffin Diet soda	None	Grilled lemon-thyme chicken breasts Risotto Vegetable antipasto Tomato & onion salad w/light olive oil & balsamic vinegar Ice milk	Ice milk
Fri.	Fresh fruit bowl Oat bran muffin Coffee w/ nonfat creamer	Tuna in water w/ balsamic vinegar Crisp bread Flavored seltzer	Decaf. w/ nonfat creamer Gingersnaps	Vegetarian pasta primavera Tri-color salad w/ low-fat dressing Melon Diet soda	None

Day of Week	Breakfast	Lunch	Afternoon Snack	Dinner	Evening Snack
Sat.	Low-fat French toast w/ syrup Turkey sausage patties Coffee w/ 1% milk Fruit juice	Cheeseburg. French fries Diet soda	Candy bar	Marinated lower-fat steak Baked potato w/ nonfat yogurt topping Asparagus w/lemon vinaigrette Lettuce & cherry tom. salad w/oil & vinegar Iced tea Fruit pie	Popcorn w/no butter at the movies
Sun.	Low-fat pancakes w/butter & syrup Bacon Fruit juice Coffee w/ 1% milk	Baked pot. w/sour cream & chives Salad bar, w/low-fat dressing	Apple Six gingersnaps	Chinese, out, w/ wonton soup Chicken w/ Chin. vegetables Yang Chow fried rice	None

Let's review Toby's meals:

Monday's breakfast is only marginally modified. Low-fat milk, low-fat margarine, and low-fat coffee creamer have been substituted for the high-fat alternatives in Toby's first eating log. At lunch (perhaps eaten in a fast-food restaurant) a grilled chicken sandwich without mayonnaise is substituted for the cheeseburger, a baked potato for the French fries. The snack changes little, except for the low-fat creamer and low-fat cookies. Toby's dinner on his original log was okay, except for the fudge cake, for which angel food cake is now substituted. The snack is still a crunchy one.

For Tuesday's breakfast, Toby was already doing pretty well. This time the fat content of the milk is lower. Toby makes certain to have healthy bread and substitutes margarine for butter. Jam, a sweet but not high-fat item, is still included. Instead of skipping lunch, Toby has a tasty, low-fat one. The Tuesday afternoon snack is dropped, part of a gradual-change process that may eventually eliminate all afternoon snacks. Dinner still focuses on meatloaf, but Toby buys low-fat ground beef, prepares the meatloaf using a low-fat recipe, and complements the loaf with low-fat foods. Dessert is a sorbet (sherbet), while the evening snack represents a complete low-fat substitution for the previous high-fat fudge cake.

Instead of skipping Wednesday breakfast, Toby has low-fat cereal, but chooses one different from his Monday choice. He may have chosen a different fruit topping as well, perhaps a canned one. Lunch still features pita bread, but this time filled with a tasty tabbouleh salad. The snack is fig bars. For dinner, Toby previously had plain broiled fish, probably not too appetizing. This time Cajun spice is the order of the day. Toby eliminates the late-night snack, as part of a gradual change aimed at reducing the frequency of that fourth meal to one or two times a week.

Thursday breakfast features scrambled eggs. (An egg is a low-calorie, relatively low-fat food. People who have to watch their cholesterol intake should use egg substitutes.) Notice he includes Canadian bacon. There are packaged Canadian bacons with only 1 to 2 grams of fat per slice. Again, with minor alterations, Toby has made a high-fat breakfast into one reasonably lower in fat. At the same time, a high-fat lunch is converted into a low-fat one. For dinner, pork chops are replaced by the second chicken dinner of the week, but the chicken is prepared in a completely different way from that eaten on Monday. Ice cream is replaced by ice milk, both for dinner dessert and late-night snack.

On Toby's original eating log, Friday was the day to be "good," one of those days many perpetual dieters observe occasionally, although the rest of their diet isn't healthy. In the current eating plan week, Friday's eating remains healthful, but is now part of a consistent program that can help Toby over time.

The fresh fruit bowl for Friday breakfast includes two to four varieties of fruit to keep it interesting. Lunch is essentially the same as it was on the original log, except that Toby has discovered balsamic vinegar, a tasty dressing that can be used without oil. Afternoon snack is unchanged. The vegetarian dinner in the original plan probably consisted of a limp collection of colorless, unappetizing stalks of this and that. This eating plan shows that more time spent in food preparation can provide a meal with a great deal of interest.

As Toby moves into the weekend, he chooses the low-fat versions of typical weekend breakfast fare. Notice also that the bacon remains on the menu for Sunday. Whether or not bacon eventually disappears from his diet, his overall eating pattern is clearly moving in the low-fat direction. Having bacon once a week will definitely not undermine the plan.

Just as a few strips of bacon each week won't sink an otherwise sound plan, neither will an occasional Saturday lunch of cheeseburger and fries eaten out with the children. And Sunday's lunch, also eaten out at a fast-food restaurant, is low fat except for the potato's sour cream topping, which he uses sparingly. Until fast-food restaurants provide nonfat baked potato toppings, try a low-fat dressing from the salad bar on your potato. You might like it.

Saturday dinner doesn't vary too much from the original log, but Toby made sure to buy a lower-fat cut of steak, the baked potato is topped with non-fat yogurt, the vegetable is a tasty one, and the fruit pie is served without the high-fat load of ice cream. Not only is the fat content of his dessert reduced, but now Toby will be able to taste the pie. Popcorn at the movies? Fine. All Toby has to do is refuse the butter. As for Sunday, here's chicken again, but this time in a low-fat Chinese restaurant dish, again providing a completely different taste. And see how easily and painlessly the rest of the meal is converted to low fat. (Yang Chow fried rice is a nongreasy version of the old staple.)

So there you have it—an eating plan gradually developed through food substitution that is healthy and tasty at the same time. In this example, most of the dishes are easy to prepare. If you like to cook, have the time, and consult one or more low-fat cookbooks (see Suggested Readings and General References), you can come up with many interesting, enticing low-fat meals to serve at home. To do that, let's go shopping the healthy way.

Let's Go Shopping

We're going to shop by aisle/section in a typical supermarket. You will, of course, set up your own shopping trip according to how products are shelved in the market you patronize.

Fruits and Vegetables

Since the produce section is almost always along an outside wall at one end of the supermarket, let's start here. Vegetables are one of the centerpieces of low-fat eating. When planning menus, you have to remember that veggies are no longer low fat if they are fried in butter, covered with a cream or cheese sauce, or coated with breading and deep-fried. Legumes (beans, peas, and lentils) are terrific low-fat foods.

Fresh fruit is also terrific as long as it is not covered with some high-fat topping. Canned fruit is also okay, as long as you don't eat the sugary syrup it's packed in. But even the sugary syrup contains no fat, so its excess calories are not as likely to be stored as body fat as the excess calories in high-fat toppings you may use now.

Breads, Cereals, and Pasta

You will probably visit these sections of the supermarket every shopping trip. This food group is central to low-fat eating, but keep in mind that commercially baked goods can be high in fat. Crackers range from low to high in fat, depending on the variety. Read labels carefully (see following). You should be able to find low-fat cookies for a snack. When buying breakfast cereal, check the label for fat content, which varies widely. Some low-fat cereals, such as some kinds of granola, are a healthy snack, too.

Meat, Poultry, and Fish

You have to be careful when shopping at this counter. The low-fat items are often outnumbered by the high-fat ones, which can be very tempting. But you don't have to eliminate meat from your diet completely. You need to cut down on total intake and eat leaner cuts. If your market provides access to its butcher, ask to have as much fat as possible trimmed from the meat you purchase. If the market doesn't offer that service, buy packaged meat and trim it yourself before cooking.

The leanest beef cuts are flank steak, tenderloin, sirloin tip, and top round. Lean pork can also be found: Canadian bacon, tenderloin, and center-cut loin chops. The only fatty veal is breaded cutlet, but chicken and turkey breasts make excellent substitutes for veal cutlets. The lean lamb cuts are loin and leg.

Poultry has fat under the skin, and if the skin is not removed, you are not buying a particularly low-fat food. Because ducks and geese are waterfowl and need protection against cold, they carry more fat under their skins than chickens and turkeys. It is possible to cook these birds for fat resolution. The skin should be removed before eating. In shopping for chicken, buy parts that have already been skinned or skin the parts yourself before cooking. If you are roasting chicken, turkey, or cornish game hen, cook it with the skin on, but remove the skin before you eat it.

With the exceptions noted in chapter 5, most varieties of fish are low in fat. However, if you are buying fish cutlets prepared with a coating, you must read the label carefully; some are high in fat. Shellfish is generally low in fat.

Milk and Other Dairy Products

You have to be as careful in the dairy department as you are at the meat counter. Obviously, not all dairy products need be eliminated to reduce the fat in your meals. But the low-fat dairy items in your supermarket are surrounded by an abundance of high-fat ones. Nevertheless, if you are selective, you can find low-fat, skim, or nonfat varieties of milk, yogurt, and cheese. Look for table cheeses with less than five grams of fat per ounce. Responding to demand, cheesemakers now produce good-tasting cheese with a fat content as low as one gram per ounce.

Buttermilk is low in fat, even though it looks and sounds fatty. In choosing nondairy substitutes (sour cream, dry creamer), read the label carefully. Make sure the product doesn't contain coconut oil. Use low-fat margarine for a butter substitute. It can be used for cooking if you heat it slowly in the frying pan.

Eggs

You won't be spending much time at the counter deciding whether to buy white or brown eggs, A or AA size, but you might decide to experiment with available egg substitutes. You may find that you like them both for use in recipes and for eating as scrambled "eggs" and omelettes.

Oils and Fats

All oil is essentially pure fat. However, some oils contain less harmful and possibly even helpful fats. Saturated fats are the most harmful. *Monounsaturated* fats (found in olive, canola, and peanut oils) and *polyunsaturated* fats may actually lower blood cholesterol. When shopping, look for monounsaturateds and oils high in polyunsaturateds: safflower, soybean, sunflower, and sesame. However, regardless of concerns about cholesterol, you want to keep your oil intake at an absolute minimum because of the high caloric content of all fats. You might want to try the nonstick vegetable oil sprays for frying. These do a good job of making your pan nonstick, and with many fewer calories than the amount of oil you'd have to use to do a similar job. Look for low-fat or nonfat salad dressings. They can be delicious.

Keeping Certain Foods Out of the Home

The primary goal of healthy food shopping is to bring healthy foods into the home; a secondary goal is to keep unhealthy foods out. You will encounter few problems if you live alone or with others who agree to join an eating program similar to yours. It becomes more complicated when there are others, especially children, who don't need or want to change the way they eat. But, low-fat eating promotes good health for everyone, and children can also learn to enjoy a moderate- to low-fat diet, if it is introduced to them *gradually* (there's that word again) and in a nonauthoritarian way. Healthy eating patterns will then be established that the children can follow their entire lives.

Try to ease children toward a low-fat diet. Still, children are children, and it will be difficult to banish cookies, cupcakes, doughnuts, and candy completely. The family may be able to consult the list of substitutes together to see if there are any mutually agreeable items that can be substituted for the foods that offend the most (giving the child some control in this situation is a good way to enlist their overall cooperation), but in the end you may have to buy some high-fat products and have them in the house.

What to do? One approach is to designate one kitchen cabinet as the storeplace for the foods you'd rather not see. You may find it easier to deal with temptation if there is only one cabinet to avoid. Ice cream in the only freezer compartment of the refrigerator is a tougher problem, for which you may need to exercise willpower. Another solution is alternating periods when foods high in refined sugar and high-fat snack foods are available at home and when they are not.

Tasty, Low-Fat Eating

Changing Tastes

Why should you take time to learn about and prepare creative low-fat dishes? We all know that veggies are healthy, but if a vegetable-based meal is not appetizing and satisfying, simply knowing that it is good for you will not be enough to offset the desire for a slice of roast beef or a chunk of cheddar. You will be inclined to choose healthier foods when the menu of your mind contains many selections of healthy dishes that you recall having enjoyed.

The most important aspect of developing a menu of appealing low-fat foods is that gradually over time you will establish new eating habits as comfortable and familiar as your current ones. High-fat foods will gradually become less appealing. Once you are committed to low-fat eating, you may find yourself wondering how you tolerated all those heavy, high-fat, high-grease meals.

Low-fat eating gives you the opportunity to rediscover colors, textures, and flavors in food that you forgot existed. Foods you never thought of eating previously may become very tempting. For example, a good bread that is fresh,

BETTER FOOD LABELS, AT LAST

It took an act of Congress, years of research, and some last-minute government wrangling. Now new nutrition labels for all processed foods will begin to appear on supermarket shelves in early 1993. All processed foods—some 300,000 varieties—must carry the new nutrition information by May 1994.

The U.S. Food and Drug Administration, which developed the labeling rules, successfully resisted food-industry pressure and held to its plan to present nutritional information as percentages of "daily values," which will help people compare different foods to see how they fit into an overall diet.

The final label format (see sample below) has several refinements over earlier drafts. Most significantly, the label lists daily values for a 2,000-calorie diet. (Earlier versions had used a 2,350-calorie diet.) The label also lists nutrient limits for a 2,500-calorie diet, useful mainly for a larger man but helpful to other consumers who want to extrapolate nutritional information for other caloric intakes.

The 2,500-calorie diet was a concession to the U.S. Department of Agriculture, which feared—along with its constituents such as cattle ranchers—that people would shun foods seemingly too high in fat in a 2,000-calorie diet. But the USDA also made significant concessions. It agreed to use the FDA's label format for any processed foods under its jurisdiction. That's a significant gain for consumers, who might otherwise have faced two different labels in the stores—one for meat lasagna (USDA), another for cheese lasagna (FDA), for example.

The FDA's daily values for fat—no more than 65 grams in a 2,000-calorie diet—equals 30 percent of calories from fat. (It might have been preferable if the government had set a limit of 25 percent.) The FDA's regulations also standardize meanings for claims: A food can't be called *light,* for example, unless it has at least 50 percent less fat than the product with which it's compared. Foods labeled "fresh" cannot have been frozen, processed, heated, or chemically preserved.

Finally, the new rules limit the labels' health hype to only a few, well-substantiated claims, such as the link between fiber and prevention of some types of cancer.

The following sample label is for a package of macaroni and cheese:

NUTRITION FACTS

Serving Size: ½ cup (114g)
Servings Per Container: 4

Amount Per Serving
Calories 260   Calories from Fat 120

	% Daily Value*
Total Fat 13g	20%
Saturated Fat 5g	25%
Cholesterol 30mg	10%
Sodium 660mg	28%
Total Carbohydrate 31g	11%
Dietary Fiber 0g	0%
Sugar 5g	
Protein 5g	

Vitamin A 4%	**Vitamin C 2%**
Calcium 15%	**Iron 4%**

Percentage of Daily Values are based on a 2,000-calorie diet. Your daily values may be higher or lower, depending on your calorie needs:

	Calories	2,000	2,500
Total Fat	Less than	65g	80g
Sat. Fat	Less than	20g	25g
Cholesterol	Less than	300mg	300mg
Sodium	Less than	2,400mg	2,400mg
Total Carbohydrate		300g	375g
Fiber		25g	30g

Calories per gram: Fat 9   Carbohydrates 4   Protein 4

Source: *Consumer Reports*, February 1993.

moist, and made with tasty low-fat ingredients can have an intriguingly light taste and texture that butter can only compromise.

Cooking Healthy

Foods don't vary that much, but meals can vary infinitely. For example, intricate Chinese cuisine can use the same combination of foods, such as chicken and Chinese vegetables, and combine them with various seasonings, preparations, coatings, sauces, slicing, and methods of cooking that can give you a month of dinners from the same basic ingredients without duplicating the same taste twice. Thus, in a low-fat eating plan, you can certainly have chicken three times a week and not be bored, provided you devote time to the planning and preparation of your meals.

Low-fat eating will be dull and uninteresting only if you let it be. It can be plain or fancy; check out the many available low-fat cookbooks (see Suggested Readings and General References). You have choices. You can make this program work if you want to, and you don't have to starve or be deprived at mealtime. The trick is to develop a repertoire of low-fat dishes so appealing that you're willing to substitute a few of them for some of the high-fat foods you are in the habit of eating. That trick has been turned countless times, and you can accomplish it too.

As you begin your adventures in low-fat eating, you will want to be sure that your diet is nutritionally balanced. The best way to do this is by following (without being compulsive about it) the food guide pyramid presented in Chart 5.1 on page 68. Now let's look at some specifics.

Vegetables. Vegetables are going to form the centerpiece of any low-fat diet you eventually adopt. Unfortunately, many people on high-fat diets seem to consider vegetables as dull, tasteless, overcooked, and mushy. So you'd better develop a passion for dull, tasteless, overcooked, mushy meals—right? Wrong, if you take time to research recipes and techniques for preparation of vegetables. Cooking time is very important to ensure that vegetables remain crisp and colorful. Follow recipe directions carefully in preparing vegetables and you will be surprised and delighted. Especially helpful in the preparation of tasty vegetables is greaseless/waterless cookware (see page 115).

Chicken. Chicken is a staple of many a low-fat diet. It can be prepared in hundreds of ways, providing perhaps as many different tastes. It appears in virtually every major cuisine. Chicken is easy to prepare and cook. Since chickens carry most of their body fat under their skin, making sure that the chicken you cook and eat is low in fat is easy to accomplish. More and more, markets offer chicken parts already skinned. However, you will find that with practice and a sharp knife skinning chicken before cooking becomes a fairly easy task. And remember, combining chicken directly with vegetables during the cooking process complements the flavors of many vegetables.

Fish. Fish is also very important to the low-fat eater and, like chicken, can be prepared in a wide variety of ways. But unlike chicken, fish comes in many types and tastes. Don't be discouraged. See variety as an opportunity to experiment, to discover for yourself the kinds of fish you like best. You can buy fish in a fish market, or frozen at the supermarket. Buy fish boned and filleted, or take care of that task yourself, either before or after cooking. Buy small fish that you will eat whole, or buy slices of large fish. Again, take time to experi-

ment with different varieties, cuts, and above all, different methods of preparation.

Meat. Why is a section on meat in a book about low-fat eating? It is a con-
firmation that you don't have to give up meat entirely, even beef, to become a
low-fat eater. There are cuts, amounts, and ways of preparation that will allow
you to retain meat in your diet. Remember, you will have to choose the low-fat
varieties, trim off all visible fat, and prepare the meat in ways that reduce the
fat as much as possible.

Salads. Salads are an important part of any low-fat diet. But not every
salad is low-fat; those that have large quantities of meat or cheese or mayonnaise, or are topped with oily or creamy dressings, usually contain plenty of fat.
Salads certainly do not have to be dull rabbit food in order to be healthy. For
example, the *American Heart Association Cookbook* lists 45 salads and 15 different dressings within 50 pages. *Low Fat and Loving It* by Ruth Spear has 6
different kinds of vinaigrette dressings, and features salads containing mushrooms, celery, black beans, corn, tomatoes, carrots, cabbage, spinach, tuna,
and wheatberries. Cuisines represented in Ruth Spear's book include Moroc-
can, Arabic, Mexican, Japanese, and Pennsylvania Dutch.

Stocks and sauces. As you become more involved with low-fat food preparation, you will find that low-fat cooking stocks and sauces can improve and
are sometimes required for many recipes. You can find sections devoted specifically to stocks and sauces in *Controlling Your Fat Tooth* by Joseph Piscatella;
the *Good Eating, Good Health Cookbook* by Phyllis Kaufman; *Gourmet Light* by
Greer Underwood; as well as Ruth Spear's *Low Fat and Loving It*.

Desserts. By now you probably realize that you do not have to forgo
scrumptious desserts to eat a low-fat diet. By substituting low-fat ingredients
for butter and cream, you can enjoy the occasional cookies, puddings, cakes,
and pies. Many examples can be found in low-fat cookbooks; one prime example is *Sumptuous Desserts the Slim Cuisine Way,* by Sue Kreitzman (Consumer
Reports Books).

Breakfast. As discussed previously, many people, especially those who
are trying to lose weight, tend to skip this essential meal. Skipping breakfast is
not a good idea, whether or not you are trying to lose weight.

Making a healthy breakfast can be either simple or complex. Easy-to-pre-
pare breakfast staples include the wide variety of low- and nonfat cold and hot
cereals (remember to read labels), fruit and fruit juices, breads and low-fat muffins with low-fat margarine and/or jam, low-fat or skim milk, low-fat cheese,
and low- or nonfat yogurt. Although fresh fruit is better than canned, you can
use the canned variety and still avoid a sugar blitz if your supermarket carries

HOW TO SHOP FOR FISH

Fish is an excellent, high-protein, low-fat food. But fish is also a product that can contain worrisome levels of hazardous chemicals and heavy metals, and can be contaminated by sloppy handling methods in stores and supermarkets.

Certain types of fish, namely salmon, swordfish, and lake whitefish, may well contain polychlorinated biphenyls (PCBs). Pregnant women, or women who expect to become pregnant, should avoid these types of fish, as should young children. Swordfish and tuna too often expose women to mercury, which could also harm a fetus. Flounder, sole, and catfish are preferable species for people in this high-risk group. Other people can pretty much eat what they like, but prudence would suggest varying the fish diet to no more than one portion a week of a food likely to contain PCBs or one likely to be high in mercury.

Here are some guidelines to follow when you are shopping for fish:

• When buying whole fish, look for bright, clear, bulging eyes. Cloudy, sunken, discolored, or slime-covered eyes signal fish that is either too old or even beginning to spoil. Avoid fish whose skin has begun to discolor, shows depressions, tears, or blemishes.

• When buying steaks or fillets, look for moist flesh that still has a translucent sheen. Watch out for flesh that's dried out or gaping (the muscle fibers are beginning to pull apart). That's a sign of over-the-hill fish.

• Note how the fish is displayed and look for clues that the storage temperature may be too high. If fish fillets are displayed inside pans surrounded by ice, that's usually a sign the retailer is paying some attention to storage practices. Whole fish should be displayed under ice.

• Carefully evaluate store specials and price reductions. Specials may be a way to move old fish.

• Look for evidence that fish has been frozen and then thawed. Chunks of ice floating in the fish liquid is a sign that the fish has been frozen. If you're not sure, ask. There's nothing wrong with frozen fish, but if you unknowingly buy fish that has already been frozen and then you refreeze it, its texture and flavor will suffer.

• Use your nose. Fresh fish smell like the sea, but they have no strong fishy odor. Strong odors usually indicate age.

unsweetened canned fruit, or if you pour off some of the syrup of sweetened fruit. If you want a more elaborate breakfast, refer to the breakfast sections of low-fat cookbooks.

Cooking Equipment

Although the first key to healthy eating is planning and choosing the right food-stuffs, the way to turn those foodstuffs into tasty and appealing meals lies in the preparation. So let's consider kitchen equipment and specific methods of cooking that can help you.

Basic cookware. A *steamer* will cook vegetables to the tenderness you want, while preserving color and flavor. And you avoid water-logged veggies, which result from cooking them directly in boiling water.

Greaseless frypans allow you to panfry foods using either no added fat or one of the low-fat cooking sprays. The low-fat cooking sprays can be used on regular cookware as well as nonstick, but the nonstick items are good investments in convenience. You may need to experiment to find the right cooking temperature so that the food will not be burned.

Greaseless/waterless cookware is far more sophisticated than greaseless fry-pans and can be purchased in various sizes and shapes. Designed for a variety of cooking tasks using no added fat, this cookware requires only a small amount of liquid to cook food. Generally made of several layers of different kinds of metal bonded together in a special way that provides even heating over the total surface area, greaseless/waterless cookware is usually more expensive than other kinds of cookware. The pans have self-sealing tops that create a semivacuum when heat is applied. In the semivacuum, foods are cooked at lower than normal temperatures; consequently, the foods themselves usually provide all or most of the moisture needed for cooking. Cleanup is very simple.

Greaseless/waterless cookware provides two different approaches to low-fat cooking. First, panbroiling meat in this cookware removes as much fat as possible. The meat cooks quickly because of the semivacuum, which also allows the retention of the meat's natural juices (it doesn't lose much moisture and doesn't shrink). This cooking method is superior to most others because it allows you to render more of the fat in beef and pork without burning or drying out the meat. And you add no fat. Low-fat cuts of meat will remain tender and juicy, an encouragement to use leaner cuts.

Second, vegetables cooked by this method are generally more colorful, crisper, and tastier than those cooked by steaming (formerly the best method of cooking vegetables). Furthermore, since the cooking temperature is around 185°F., a much higher proportion of the nutrients and vitamins in the vegetables are preserved than is the case with either boiling or steaming, both of which cook at 212°F. or above.

A *microwave oven* cooks faster and with less fuss than the other cooking systems, and it also reduces vitamin loss. Microwave ovens are commonly used for boiling coffee water, microwaving a potato (although the crisp skin many devoted baked potato lovers cannot do without is lost), or reheating leftovers. However, if you take some time and pay careful attention to recipes and instructions about proper microwave use, you should be able to master complicated cooking tasks and produce dishes more elaborate than baked potatoes. Many cookbooks are devoted to microwave cooking. Combine the information from the cookbooks with what you now know about low-fat eating and food shopping, and you can become a very effective low-fat cook, using the microwave almost exclusively.

A *wok* allows you to prepare stir-fried vegetables using only small amounts of the healthier cooking oils such as olive or peanut. The wok's advantage over the steamer is that you season the vegetables while they cook and can add meat, poultry, shellfish, or fish directly to the mixture, interlacing flavors to make the final result more distinctive. Many Asian cuisines use the wok as the primary cooking implement, and many cookbooks are available to provide recipes for wok cooking. As with microwave cooking, you need to spend some time learning how to use the wok correctly.

An *automatic bread-making machine* allows you to whip up a variety of delicious, low-fat breads without too much effort. Again, you must spend some time learning how to use the machine. Always use low-fat bread recipes—an extensive selection can be found in the *American Heart Association Cookbook*—or substitute low-fat ingredients in standard recipes. Some special skill needs to be developed, because changing the combination of ingredients in any bread may alter the rate at which it rises.

Utensils. A *food processor* or *blender* is very helpful for making various dressings, dips, toppings, and drinks that are based on nonfat yogurt.

A *bulb baster* simplifies removal of fat from gravies and sauces.

A *gravy separator* can help drain nonfat juices from meat drippings.

Sharp knives and *poultry shears* are helpful for trimming visible fat from meat and removing poultry skin before cooking.

Organizing Your Kitchen

Placing all your cooking utensils and equipment within easy reach can be another important key to making low-fat cooking a welcome and convenient part of your day.

First organize your kitchen so that you have adequate work surfaces and storage areas. If possible, store the various recipe components near the places you intend to prepare and cook them. If you need more work and/or storage space, try to create it by rearrangement, rather than extension or renovation.

Develop a schedule, allowing time for preparation, cooking, and, if necessary, cooling. It's sometimes easier to prevent messes than clean them up. If possible, clean up as you work, put ingredient containers away after you use them, and rinse or wash mixing bowls and/or place them in the dishwasher as soon as you are through with them.

Healthy Cooking Methods

Meat. Cook meat by methods that eliminate as much fat as possible: pan-broil in greaseless/waterless cookware; roast at medium heat (around 325°F.) and use a rack to keep the meat out of its drippings; roast in a covered pot with a nonfat liquid such as lemon juice added before cooking; braise (roasting in flavored liquid, after first searing all sides); sauté (cook at high temperature in a frying pan) but stir the meat or other food constantly so that virtually no cooking oil is needed; stir-fry (an Asian version of sautéing, grilling, or broiling); poach (immerse and barely cover food in a simmering layer of cooking liquid).

If you prepare meat the day before you plan to serve it, refrigerate it after cooking and remove any congealed fat before reheating. If you use ground beef, sauté it and then place it on paper towels to drain the fat. Use smaller portions of meat—as a condiment instead of a main course. For example, in preparing a dinner for four, rather than serve each guest an individual steak, slice one steak very thin and mix it with vegetables for four in a stir-fry dish.

Chicken. There is virtually no fat in chicken, turkey, and other poultry muscle, but there is plenty of fat under the skin. And fat is added by many traditional methods of preparing chicken, such as frying or covering it with gravy. Don't use fat when cooking poultry. Use a nonstick pan and/or a cooking spray when cooking on top of the stove, and try roasting, broiling, grilling, or poaching. Remember to remove the skin prior to eating.

As noted previously, chicken franks and other prepared poultry cuts are not necessarily low in fat. The liquid used in most self-basting turkey preparations is fairly high in fat. Ground turkey can also be very fatty. Check the labels carefully.

Fish. Like poultry, fish can become a high-fat food if not cooked properly. Don't bread and deep-fry it. Don't panfry it in butter, or margarine. Fry fish in a nonstick pan with a small amount of cooking spray, or grill, broil, or poach it. Baking fish in a small amount of wine is also good.

Vegetables. Avoid boiling. Although boiling doesn't add fat, it destroys color, texture, taste, and nutrients. Preparation in greaseless/waterless cookware produces vegetables that look and taste superb. Steaming and stir-frying are also good methods of cooking vegetables. Broiling on a skewer, with or without meat or chicken, can produce tasty results, as can baking and roasting. Microwaving is another cooking method that suits both fresh and frozen vegetables. It's quick, and most important, helps retain the essential vitamins and minerals. As you are aware, many vegetables can be eaten raw, with or without dressing; try serving them with tasty dip made from nonfat yogurt.

Cooking Aids

There are several classes of cooking aids to use in your low-fat cooking program.

Lubricants. When the dish you are preparing requires lubrication, use a small amount of vegetable oil, a low-fat nonstick spray, wine, lemon juice, wine or herb vinegar, a low-fat broth (see the stock section of any low-fat cookbook), or water. Since cuts of meat lower in fat are generally less tender than fattier ones, consider marinating them overnight before cooking. Most low-fat cookbooks have one or more marinade recipes. Olive oil, used sparingly, is good for panfrying, but of course its special taste must complement the food you are cooking. A thin layer of a nonfat liquid such as wine or diluted lemon juice can be used in a frying pan as the lubricant, so long as you replace the liquid as it evaporates. If salt intake is not a problem for you, try a small amount of soy sauce.

Seasonings. Learn how to use herbs and spices creatively. Dry mustard and curry powder, sprinkled on while cooking, are easy to use and fun to taste. Fresh hot pepper, used sparingly until you are used to it, can spice up many bland vegetables such as mushrooms and string beans. Garlic works wonders too, but to avoid unpleasantness at home maybe everyone should eat it the same day. Grated citrus peel makes a great flavoring, as do citrus juice and vinegar (added at the last minute). Dried mushrooms, tomatoes, and raisins add flavor to many dishes. The *American Heart Association Cookbook* has an excellent and detailed seasoning guide for those who want to learn more about the world of seasonings.

7

Exercise

First Thoughts

"Oh, yuck!" may be your first reaction when you contemplate exercise. If so, you are in the majority. In fact, if you need to be on Pathway C to weight loss, you may be particularly discouraged, or even depressed, to know that regular exercise represents your last, best chance to escape the yo-yo dieting cycle. Even if you're on Pathway A or B and know that exercise may not be essential to weight loss, you have to concede that it will contribute a great deal to your prospects for long-term success.

Weight-Loss Benefits of Exercise

The first benefit is that your body will have to tap stored fat if your food intake doesn't supply the additional calories needed to meet the new energy requirements created by exercise. Second, exercise will raise a previously depressed resting metabolic rate (RMR); it does this by creating new muscle, which requires more energy for daily sustenance than fat. Stimulating muscle development also avoids another weight-loss pitfall—loss of muscle mass that accompanies many calorie-restriction diets. Last, exercise increases the ability of muscles to store excess carbohydrate as glycogen (the body's storage form of carbohydrate) rather than converting it into stored fat.

Common Problems of Exercise

Regular exercise presents several problems that are shared by many overweight and nonoverweight people alike. The most common problem is, of course, not exercising at all. Another is exercising in fits and starts, with neither consistency nor regularity. Then there is overdoing it, which can lead to musculoskeletal pain and even injury. Finally, there is the universal complaint that exercise is no fun.

It's Not the Exercise, It's the Regularity

For many people, the toughest aspect to deal with in becoming a regular exerciser is the regularity, not the exercise. As you begin this project, your first objective should be to prepare yourself to set aside the time you are going to need for your program. A commitment to regular exercise that will in fact be regular requires thinking through what you intend to do and the time it will require, then thinking about it some more, and finally reaching a decision you can accept.

The particular form your exercise takes is not important at this point. It can be walking for 10 minutes or so, three times a week, for a couple of weeks—just plain walking at your regular pace. Your focus should not be on the exercise itself, but on the *habit* of exercising. You must consciously reinforce that whatever your other obligations may be, this special time—first thing in the morning, just after the kids are off to school, on your lunch break, or before or after dinner—has been scheduled for yourself.

Happily, once you begin to follow an exercise schedule, even a few times for short periods, you will probably find that you begin to feel better. Why? It's not that your body is changing, at least not so soon; it's that your mental attitude has started to change. You have begun to take control, to take responsibility. You have added a new life experience, something novel and different, something that's going to help you achieve goals you want to achieve for yourself—knowing this is certain to give you a good feeling.

At the beginning, don't concern yourself about speed, time, or distance traveled. Placing yourself on a regular schedule is enough challenge for a previously sedentary person or a long-lapsed exerciser. Once you establish a regular schedule, you will go longer, farther, faster soon enough.

The Intrusiveness of Regular Exercise

It is unavoidable that becoming a regular exerciser will intrude upon the established patterns of your life and, if your objective is to maintain your weight at a new, lower level, the intrusion will likely continue for the rest of your life. You must recognize, accept, and adjust to it. Of all the life-style and behavioral changes you can undertake to improve your health—abstaining from tobacco or drug use, changing your eating habits, wearing your automobile seat belt—

only exercise requires a permanent commitment of time. In comparison, smokers and problem drinkers who have decided to stop may spend some time in therapy, cessation classes, or support groups, but these are time-limited experiences. For most people, once the classes or support groups end, the new behavior will no longer cost time, and, indeed, often provides a dividend of time. Not so with exercise.

To be a regular exerciser, you must be prepared to reserve time in your schedule far into the future. It may be only two or three hours per week for the exercise itself, plus another hour or two changing clothes, showering, or traveling to a pool or gym. But you will be devoting those three to six hours *each week* to your exercise program.

You should carefully examine this aspect of the project. How do you spend your time now? Do you spend many hours a week watching television? This one is easy—if exercising costs you four hours a week of TV viewing, you will be rejuvenating your mind as well as your body. But if you don't have a block of time you can take from TV, can you plan to get up 45 minutes earlier four days a week (including weekends) and reduce wasted time by 15 minutes each of those days? Can you get your spouse to help with household chores such as food shopping and cooking? Can you find time during the workday to exercise? Better yet, can you take advantage of the exercise programs that many employers now sponsor?

For most weeks of the Take Control Exercise Plan training schedules (see chapter 8), one-half or more of the total time is during the weekends. This may make it easier for you. Still, weekdays or weekends, most people can find the time if they want to. But you have to plan, and you have to take control.

Aerobic and Nonaerobic Exercise

Aerobic is a word coined and popularized in its modern sense during the 1960s by Dr. Kenneth Cooper. Aerobic exercise uses oxygen intake as its primary energy source. In contrast, the energy source for the other kind of exercise, anaerobic, is a chemical already inside the muscles. *Anaerobic* exercise, such as that done by sprinters, can be done very fast, but not for very long. Aerobic exercise can be done for very long periods of time, but not as fast. Aerobic exercise also means that your muscles are using more oxygen than they normally do.

Many people who exercise on a regular basis do it aerobically. If you choose to exercise aerobically, you will gain more weight-loss benefits in terms of using excess calories and elevating your resting metabolic rate (RMR) over a shorter period of time. *But remember that exercise doesn't have to be aerobic to contribute to weight loss.* Any increase in muscular activity above your normal levels will burn extra calories and help raise a depressed RMR. Actually, if you haven't exercised in a long time, you don't want to begin by elevating your heart rate to heights it's seldom achieved.

A Broad Range of Suitable Activities and Sports

Most people trying to establish an exercise program for themselves begin with ordinary walking, not with a sport. When you reach a point of engaging in a sport, one key to success will be choosing one that is right for you—one with which you are comfortable, which you enjoy, and which you are capable of doing. No one exercise is ideal for everyone, no one sport is better for all people.

The list of popular activities begins with aerobic walking, referred to in this book as *pace walking* (see chapter 9). In addition, there are running; cycling (indoors and out); swimming (in a pool and in open water); rowing (on open water or indoors on a machine); cross-country skiing (outdoors on snow and indoors on a machine); jumping rope; running or walking indoors on a tread-mill; roller skating; indoor running in place, on a trampoline, or a track; and stair-climbing on a machine.

Other popular activities include aerobic dance and its many variants—high- and low-impact, stepping, and jazzercise. You can do them on your own at home, with your own music tapes or a commercial video, or with one of the many televised workout sessions; you can also join an organized class at a health club. If you have the skills and enjoy competition in your workout, you might try racket sports: tennis, racket ball, and squash. Racket sports can be aerobic for you if you play singles and don't stand around between rallies. If you like competitive team sports, full-court basketball can be aerobic for you too. Furthermore, you don't have to limit yourself to doing one sport at a time. *Cross-training,* that is, doing two or more sports concurrently in a regular program, has many advantages (see chapter 8).

The most important point is that you choose an activity or sport and follow it according to your plan. If you decide after a reasonable trial that you have made the wrong choice, don't give up and go back to your old sedentary ways—try another. If that one isn't right, try another. Given the broad range of physical activities available, almost everyone should be able to find one that will be both valuable and enjoyable.

First Steps

Setting Goals and Objectives

As we discussed earlier in this book, setting goals is the foundation for success. What do you want to accomplish? Do you want to lose weight? Lose fat? Become fit? Look better? Feel better physically? Feel better about yourself? Reduce your disease risk? All of the above? Why? For yourself, for someone else, or for another reason? Remember, you will be able to follow your plan only if your motivation comes from within. If you are exercising in response to external pressures, you will more likely reap a harvest of anger, guilt, frustration, and injury than of happy, healthy, gradual, comfortable, and permanent weight and fat loss.

Think about your exercise goals and how to accomplish them. You should also think about reasonable goals and objectives in the sport you may have chosen. You now have two goals and objectives to think about: those for your weight-loss program and those for your exercise program.

Perhaps you have decided to pace walk; consider these hypothetical goals and objectives. Your first objectives may be to pace walk 20 minutes without stopping, three times a week. You may set an intermediate objective of pace walking a mile without stopping. It is important to keep in mind when formulating next-stage objectives that they should be reasonably within your reach. If you are now sedentary you will not become successful by setting an unattainable goal, such as running a marathon, as your first exercise objective. However, that goal may be possible if you enter the world of exercise slowly, carefully, and gradually.

Consistency and Regularity

Establishing consistency and regularity are two important keys to your success as a regular exerciser, both for resetting your RMR upward and for continuing to improve your fitness level. The term *fitness* applies both to musculoskeletal fitness, which allows you to do increased physical work over time using one or more major muscle groups, and to cardiovascular fitness, the increasing ability of the heart over time to beat faster and pump more blood with each beat, within the limits of healthy functioning.

Consistency refers to the length of individual training sessions. Most aerobic exercisers want to achieve both musculoskeletal and cardiovascular fitness, goals that cannot be achieved if the lengths of your training sessions vary widely. Research in exercise physiology has shown that the body does not respond well to an erratic approach. A lack of consistency in an exercise program seldom leads to progress in either kind of fitness, and it increases the risk of both injury and illness.

If you plan to increase the lengths of your training sessions, do so gradually. For example, if you are in Phase II or III of the Take Control Exercise Plan (see chapter 8) and the schedule calls for two hours per week, follow the recommended distribution of time among the training sessions as closely as possible. Don't try doing a 10-minute session, then 40, then 70. Keep to a consistent schedule, if possible.

Regularity concerns the distribution of training sessions during the week and the distribution of workout weeks over the course of a year. Consider that the Phase III Maintenance Program (see Table 8.4, page 151) requires an average total of two hours a week exercise time. You could meet this objective by doing two 60-minute training sessions, one each on Saturday and Sunday. However, this approach will benefit neither your heart nor your metabolism nearly as much as a more regular distribution of training sessions. Exercising heavily only on the weekends, at which times you boost your heart rate to a high of perhaps 85 percent of your theoretical maximum, could actually be harmful. Such intermittent spurts of accelerated heart rate could increase your risk of sudden death from heart attack.

An uneven distribution of training sessions may also wreak havoc on your musculoskeletal system. Muscles exercised regularly, at least once every other day, go through a gradual cycle of buildup, breakdown, and further buildup, which leads to increased strength and endurance over time. However, muscles that are worked only intermittently will hurt after those intermittent training sessions but will not develop increased strength and endurance.

Protecting Yourself Against Injury and Illness

Preparing for regular exercise. If you have been sedentary for some time, before you start you should follow the recommendations in chapter 4 concerning a medical checkup. If you have an illness such as coronary artery disease (heart attack or angina) or chronic lung disease, you must discuss your exercise plans with your physician. Do not delay going to your doctor because you fear that he or she will forbid you to exercise. Many doctors now recognize that regular exercise with proper medical supervision can be helpful in the management of several illnesses, provided the patient respects certain constraints. The results of tests that your doctor can perform will reveal much information about which exercises you can do safely, how strenuously you can perform them, and what signs you should be alert for as you exercise.

Taking care of your heart. Whether or not you have a history of heart-related ailments, check with your doctor if you experience any pain or unusual feelings in your chest or arms that do not seem to be related to specific muscles you may have stressed during your exercise.

Preventing injuries. Exercise-related injuries can be classified into two groups: intrinsic and extrinsic. *Intrinsic* injury comes from doing the exercise or sport. Most common are overuse injuries—shin splint, swimmer's shoulder, tennis elbow, and stress fracture of the leg. *Extrinsic* injury results from collision with a physical obstacle—an automobile, a pothole, a dangling tree branch, another exerciser, or a strolling mother and child.

The key to avoiding intrinsic injury is never to overuse your muscles. The key to avoiding extrinsic injury is to be alert to your changing surroundings—road surface, traffic, all potential obstacles. Cycling outdoors requires an especially high level of alertness.

You need proper equipment for most aerobic sports. Shoe design, fit, quality, and degree of wear are critical for avoiding overuse injury (see chapter 9). For sports in which bad technique can quickly lead to injury, you must learn good technique and use it. You must pay attention to safety rules in sports such as cycling and swimming. A very important element in injury prevention is to make sure that your training sessions do not take you too far, too fast, too often.

Overuse injuries are common in running and high-impact aerobic dance and can occur in several other aerobic sports, especially where the sport sometimes controls the participant. Dr. Kenneth Cooper, who coined the word *aerobic,* states that anyone who runs more than 15 to 20 miles (about two-and-a-half to three hours for the average runner) each week is doing it for reasons other than health. You will receive increasing *fitness* benefits by running up to about 75 miles a week, but no increased *health* benefits. Since the mid-1980s when 120 to 140 miles a week were in vogue for top runners, even some of the world-class marathoners have cut down their mileage, and have been including other aerobic sports in their training programs.

Pace walking has a very low risk of overuse injury. Nevertheless, virtually all the risks of any regular aerobic exercise can be either minimized or entirely eliminated by taking reasonable precautions.

Stress. Regular exercise should help you to manage stress in your life better. Exercise should certainly not cause stress. Cut down on the amount and intensity of your training if you find that your exercise program induces stress. By becoming a regular exerciser, you are taking control of an important part of your life. At the same time, you must be careful not to let the exercise take control of you. Remember that balance is not only the key to health but also is the key to healthy exercise.

Drink plenty of water. Remaining adequately hydrated is one of the most important injury prevention measures you can take in any sport that causes you to sweat. (You can even become overheated if you swim vigorously in warm water.) In hot weather, it is especially important to drink enough water, regardless of the sport you are doing. And this means *drinking water before you are thirsty.* Because of the way the body's low-hydration detection mechanism works, if you wait until you are thirsty, it may be too late and you may be at risk for heat exhaustion, sunstroke, or worse. On a hot day, if you find your mouth feeling very dry, stop and drink plenty of fluids before starting out again. If you are also feeling unusually warm or have a headache or find yourself a bit disoriented, get out of the sun and, if at all possible, get a ride back to your starting point.

Making Exercise Fun

For many people who contemplate a regular exercise program, the first and most important question is either "Will it be fun?" or "Won't it be a bore?" Some people think, This is going to be terrible. I'm going to hate it every step of the way, but I've got to do it. I've got to get in shape. But exercise often turns out to be fun even for those with negative attitudes, and within a couple of weeks, they are enjoying themselves. So if you go into it with a positive attitude, and consider some of the following suggestions and advice, your chances of exercising comfortably and enjoyably will significantly increase.

Rhythm. Most of the sports you will be doing—pace walking, running, cycling, swimming, aerobic dance, rowing—are served by and require a sense of rhythm. You may find this aspect of your sport enjoyable for the innate delight it provokes. Letting a natural sense of rhythm mark your movements will help you find a flow, a feeling of being in control of your body. As you exercise, move rhythmically and breathe rhythmically. Too much of what we do in life is without rhythm; exercise is rhythmic—enjoy it.

Weather. If the sport you choose takes you outdoors, you may develop or deepen your appreciation of the changing seasons. A run or a pace walk on a sunny, cold, crisp winter day can be invigorating. Summertime is great for those who like working up a sweat under that energy machine called the sun. Many people think that the best seasons for outdoor exercise are spring and fall, when the sun is shining and the temperature is moderate. Remember to dress properly, don't try to go too fast, and make sure that you can get enough water to drink.

Thinking. Many people most enjoy regular exercise when they learn to use their training sessions for thinking. You can plan your day while you work out in the morning, or review your day while you work out in the evening. Think about projects, problems, or triumphs; your exercise time provides you with time to sort things out with no phone calls, no interruptions from family or co-workers. One caveat: Safety requires that if you choose cycling, you must focus first on the road.

Routes. If you become a pace walker, cyclist, or a runner you may find one favorite route to follow over and over again. On the other hand, variety can help maintain your interest. You can also add variety by using different routes in your neighborhood, routes with different challenges. If you are a cyclist, you can select one hilly ride, another that is flat, and a longer combination route. As you become more involved in your Take Control Exercise Plan, you will need to develop routes of different distances.

Companions. One of the best ways to deal with boredom during your training sessions is to include a companion. There is nothing like conversation to help a workout session pass quickly. If the buddy system appeals to you, you must find the right partner. You will need someone with whom you can establish a regular schedule and who works out at a similar pace. This person should be someone with whom you have a lot in common and with whom you can have stimulating conversations. Probably the most realistic solution is someone with whom you would feel comfortable only occasionally, so you'll be able to retain some of your exercise time for yourself.

You might also look for a companion in one of the walking, running, or cycling clubs in your area. No such club? Start one (see Appendix D).

Some people find that dogs are the ideal companions. Conversation is one-way and you don't have to talk when you don't feel like it. Dogs can generally keep up with you and usually have as much stamina as people, yet unlike human companions dogs never need to prove they have more. Of course you have to train dogs to understand that regular exercising and dog-walking are two different enterprises. Your dog must be trained to recognize that stopping at fire hydrants and lampposts, getting acquainted with other dogs, and sniffing the neighborhood's most compelling odors are appropriate only for dog-walking, not exercising. Once you accomplish this training, your dog will generally trot along at your pace.

Listening to music. Many people deal with potential boredom by listening to music, talk radio, or other electronic distractions while they work out. A wide variety of radios and tape players are available to use while running, pace walking, indoor cycling and rowing, stair-climbing, or even swimming. A variety of belts and pouches carry electronics comfortably. Also available are audio tapes with rhythmic music played at various cadences.

A headset can be a great distraction while exercising, for good or bad. When you are exercising outdoors you must be able to hear as well as see potential danger. In the interest of safety, you must have your ears open to the outside world so that you can receive warning of impending problems such as an automobile rapidly approaching from behind. Never use the plug-in-the-ear kind of headset. Use only the airflow type with the small sponge, or the mini-speakers that stand perpendicular to the sides of your head. Never put earphones, even the airflow type, directly over your ears. If you place them on the bone directly in front of your ears, you will hear plenty via bone conduction. Never play music too loudly; it's unsafe and could damage your hearing.

Never listen to music while bicycling outdoors. Of all aerobic exercisers, cyclists are most prone to injury from external causes—automobiles, people, animals, other cyclists, and road conditions. For safety, you must concentrate fully on your route. If you find cycling boring, choose another sport rather than trying to solve the problem by listening to music.

Setting nonexercise-related goals. Sometimes adding an errand to a training session can help you relieve bordeom. Plan to pick up your newspaper, a container of milk, or a loaf of bread while you are out on your training session. Do your post office business as part of some sessions. If your car needs servicing, leave the car and bike, run, or pace walk home. When the car is ready to be picked up, reverse the sequence. If you are single, and live in area where aerobic exercisers congregate, joining that group can be a good way to meet new people. City parks are ideal venues for this purpose.

Rewards. Reward yourself for performance measured in weeks of exercise, total time, distance, or increased speed. Rewards can be clothing, special foods, a new or treasured experience, or a piece of much-needed equipment. Self-rewarding takes discipline because nothing prohibits you from indulging in rewards even if you fail to meet your exercise objective. But if you can delay the reward until you have completed a particular portion of your Take Control Exercise Plan, you will help make regular exercise fun.

Travel. If work takes you to other cities, you will have opportunities to add more interest to your exercise. Try to plan some time for at least one training session in each city on your itinerary. The following list suggests only a few of the interesting places around the United States:

• Central Park in New York City's borough of Manhattan. Circling the reservoir in the northern half of the park is a 1.6-mile cinder path, a protected place to pace walk or run. The park drives provide varied routes up to 6-plus miles in length for running, pace walking, cycling, and roller skating. The drives are open to vehicular traffic only during weekday rush hours, and even then one lane is reserved for pedestrians and exercisers.

• Prospect Park in Brooklyn reserves a lovely 3.4-mile loop of park drive for walkers, runners, and cyclists during most daylight hours of the week.

• The Trinity Trail, which runs for miles along the banks of the Trinity River in Fort Worth, Texas, is open to walkers, runners, and cyclists. This path is quiet, smooth, and has no vehicular traffic.

• The Parkway is a broad boulevard in Philadelphia that leads from the business district to the Museum of Fine Arts. There you can climb the steps with the words of the "Rocky" theme playing in your head and stop at the statue of Philadelphia's most famous fictional character, Rocky Balboa. You can then proceed to a winding, tree-lined path along the Schuylkill River.

• Chicago's Lake Front provides several miles of flat paths for running or pace walking in sight of the famous skyline.

• Washington's federal area offers many miles of flat paths with vistas of the Potomac, our national monuments, and government buildings. You can find paths across gentle hills in Rock Creek Park.

• Along the banks of Boston's Charles River are miles of protected pathways for pace walkers, runners, and cyclists.

Competitive sports. People who enjoy competition and possess reasonably special athletic skills often choose racket sports and team sports such as basketball. If you engage in these sports primarily as part of an aerobic exercise program, you must make sure that you do them aerobically. For example, aerobic tennis requires you to be a reasonably skilled player, to play against people who are at least as good as you, and to play singles with a lot of running. It is easier to maintain an aerobic level in squash or racket ball than in tennis, as long as neither player spends a lot of time standing around at change of service.

The major disadvantage of competitive sports is that they require prearranged appointments with one or more other people and court space, which usually has to be reserved in advance. Again, you might think about a competitive sport as only one component of a multisport program.

Racing. If you are doing one or more of the endurance sports, you might consider racing. Many running and walking races offer separate competitions defined by the entrant's age. You don't have to worry about being humiliated by your lack of world-class speed, because many entrants in any road race are in it only to have a good time.

There are two major reasons you might want to try racing. First, races are fun. You often meet interesting people, many accompanied by a cheering section of family and friends. The highest hopes of most entrants are to complete the course and maybe set a new personal best for themselves. Very few participate with hope of winning; as a result, there is little competitiveness. Most often there is a big group of fun-loving people out to have a good time, running or walking as fast as they can on that particular day.

Second, racing can provide a focus for your training, which can help alleviate the potential boredom of your regular sessions. You can schedule a series of events that break up the training year or session into manageable blocks of time. If you are interested in racing, see Appendix C for details on how to get started.

You may not like the competitiveness of road racing or would rather not walk in a race that's primarily for runners; however, if you have organizational skills and time to devote to an interesting project, see Appendix D for a guide to establishing noncompetitive pace walking races.

Where to Exercise

You can exercise outdoors, indoors at home, or at a club. Each has its advantages and disadvantages. The location is in part determined by the sport(s) you choose.

Outdoors. A wide variety of exercises can be done outdoors, from walking to cycling to sculling. The most common outdoor exercises are walking, pace walking, jogging, and running. If any of these are your choices, you can do them all anywhere you can walk. But some locations are more pleasant, comfortable, and safer than others.

If you are participating in a foot sport on pavement, blacktop is preferable to concrete; the former offers some slight resilience, the latter none. You should walk on pavement instead of dirt paths. To avoid injury on dirt paths you must really concentrate on the walking surface, and this can interfere with your enjoyment. Concentrating on the walk and your surroundings is much more pleasant and productive.

In general, the best places to walk or run in cities are parks, which usually offer pleasant visual surroundings that make your workouts more enjoyable. If certain paths or roadways within the park are set aside for walkers and runners and, if the roadways are wide enough to provide safety, cyclists can have a continuous stretch of pavement with no need to worry about vehicular traffic. You will often encounter some hills, usually not too steep, which present a challenge and add variety. Parks with provisions for exercise attract exercisers, so you will almost always have company when working out. Pathways along waterfronts, whether part of a park system or not, are usually conducive to a good workout.

Lightly trafficked streets in suburban neighborhoods are also good; the pavement is usually smooth blacktop. Pleasant surroundings provide stimulation and relaxation at the same time. To be safe, walk facing traffic. In most suburbs you can usually find a school track for your workout. Most schools make their tracks available for public use except during after-school practice hours, and suburban school tracks usually have good surfaces. The only problem with pace walking or running on a track is boredom, which can be alleviated by working out with a partner. Country roads and lanes also offer a nice venue for running or pace walking, assuming the pavement is acceptable.

Living in a city that does not have a park with a suitable path presents problems. Joining a fitness center that has an indoor track is one solution. However, after you have walked or run around the track a thousand times you may find it boring. The problems presented by city streets can be overcome, but you must be very attentive to your surroundings, the condition of the pavement, traffic, other pedestrians, and traffic signals. Use the sidewalk to be safe. If you have no other choice but to walk or run in the street, be careful, and go slowly until you are comfortable maneuvering around, through, and over the many obstacles you encounter.

Indoors at home. Many sports can be done indoors at home, such as pace walking or jogging on a treadmill, cycling on an indoor bike, and doing aerobic dance using instructions from a television show or video. Exercise at home has many advantages:

You need no extra time to reach your workout place.

You don't have to worry about the weather.

You can play the music you prefer, as loud as you wish, if you are home alone.

Indoor workouts are usually safe if you deal with potential hazards, such as children or pets underfoot and slippery rugs.

You can place a treadmill, indoor bike, or other machine in front of a television set.

You can use a reading stand while cycling on an indoor bike.

Health clubs. If a health club is convenient and affordable and has the equipment and facilities you want, it can be a fun place to work out because other people are usually there. Also, the better clubs provide facilities you cannot duplicate at home or find easily elsewhere: an indoor track, a swimming pool, and complete sets of controlled weight machines. A staff is usually available to help you learn to use the equipment and to design a program of exercise that will work for you (see chapter 9).

Exercising Safely

When to work out. No one time during the day is right for everyone; it is really a matter of preference and what time is best for your schedule. Because exercise promotes the secretion of the hormone insulin to mobilize energy-supplying glycogen from the liver making you feel less hungry, working out before dinner may be the best for weight loss (if cutting down on caloric intake is part of your Pathway Down). Many people prefer to work out before breakfast; morning workouts often provide a psychological lift that lasts all day. If your workplace has changing facilities and showers, you may find lunchtime workouts to be effective. Exercising outdoors at night is not recommended, except along brightly lit streets or roads in crime-free neighborhoods. Many parks are unsafe at night, even when other people are there. Even if you dress in reflective clothing and always walk or run facing traffic, you increase your risk of injury if you use a dark road at night.

Be aware. One of the great pleasures of aerobic exercise is the opportunity to get away, alone with your thoughts. Some runners report feeling so peaceful and calm they become unaware they are running. Unless you are working out in an isolated place, shutting out the real world can be dangerous. You should always maintain some level of awareness of your surroundings and be alert for potential problems.

Keep your head up. Many of us tend to look squarely at the ground while engaging in a footsport. It is a good idea to check the pavement occasionally for danger, but you must also look ahead of yourself for that overhanging branch, big pothole, puddle of leftover rainwater, fallen power line, or angry dog. Note cars that are being driven erratically, backed out of driveways, or are turning onto the road in your direction. To avoid a collision on a park roadway heavily used by cyclists, walk opposite the direction that most of them ride.

8

The Take Control

Exercise Plan

GET READY

The Take Control Exercise Plan* is designed for use by regular exercisers at any level, from beginner to athlete. The program will help a beginner ease into regular exercise, as gradually and painlessly as possible. If you are a more experienced sportsperson, the exercise plan should provide a sufficiently challenging, yet comfortable program, one that will keep you in shape without pushing you to overdo it. While rigorous in its demand for consistency and regularity, the plan retains an internal flexibility that allows you to move around from high-volume weeks to low-volume weeks, depending on your needs and level of fitness. As with the Take Control Eating Plan, the choices are yours.

The Principles

The Take Control Exercise Plan is based on an approach to sports training developed by Bill Bowerman, the world-renowned middle-distance running coach from the University of Oregon. Bowerman set out 10 basic principles to train athletes for many competitive events. The following 7 are adapted for use in the Take Control Exercise Plan:

1. Training must be regular, according to a long-term plan.
2. Moderation is the watchword.

*As noted in chapter 4, if you have any of the eight diseases or conditions listed on page 54, a medical checkup and physician's clearance is recommended before you start any exercise program. Otherwise, if you follow the gradual-change approach, there should be little health risk in becoming a regular exerciser, although the risk in engaging in any vigorous activity or exertion can never be fully eliminated.

3. The workload must be balanced; overtraining, which can lead to fatigue, injury, and loss of motivation, must be avoided.
4. You must know your goals and they must be realistic ones.
5. Training schedules should be planned with a hard/easy rotation, both from day to day and more generally over time.
6. Rest should be scheduled regularly.
7. Working out should be fun, whenever possible.

Consider these principles for a moment. Incorporating them into your thinking will help establish you as a regular exerciser.

Phases of the Take Control Exercise Plan

The Take Control Exercise Plan has three phases: introduction, development, and maintenance. Each lasts 13 weeks.

The first, your introduction to regular exercise, requires three workouts each week.

The second develops your skills and abilities as a Take Control exerciser. It enables you to begin building strength and endurance, the primary physical requirements for successful ongoing regular exercise. This phase requires four workouts each week.

The third phase offers three levels of maintenance. The first level has an every-other-day schedule, three days one week, four days the next. The second level has a four-day-a-week schedule, and the third level has five days. You can pick one level to stay with, alternate between two of them, or rotate among all three.

As you can see, you incorporate the exercise plan into your daily schedule as you did the eating plan: Change habits gradually; take small, nontaxing steps into your new life; and solidify gains at one step before you go on to the next.

Forward-Motion and In-Place Activities and Sports

Physical activities and sports (see chapter 9) can be conveniently divided into two groups, forward motion and in-place. Forward-motion sports include pace walking, running, swimming, bicycling, rowing, and other activities that were traditionally associated with the outdoors. However, most forward-motion activities can now be performed indoors if you have the right equipment and venue. In many instances, these activities can become in-place sports.

In-place activities and sports include aerobic dance, stepping, weight training, and stair-climbing. Because these activities require little space they are more easily done indoors.

If you have not exercised regularly in some time, walking (graduating eventually to pace walking) is a very good activity with which to reintroduce yourself to regular exercise. It does not risk injury to your undertrained muscles and spares your joints the shocks of the sudden onset of a running program. You will find that walking is most pleasantly relaxing . Walking is the ideal way to begin exercising, whether you intend to try forward motion or an in-place sport/activity, or are thinking about a program that includes two or more sports at the same time (see the section on pace training on pages 153–54), or even if you haven't yet made up your mind about what you are going to do for exercise.

However, it is your program and perhaps you would rather begin your exercise plan doing aerobic dance at home in front of the TV for 10 minutes at a time. Or you may prefer going to a gym to exercise slowly on the stair climber. That's fine too. Remember as you read this chapter that the suggested programs are only guides. You are in control and will decide how to begin your program.

Minutes Not Miles

Take Control workouts should be measured in minutes not miles, whether you engage in forward motion or in-place sports or activities. If you choose forward-motion sports, you need not be concerned with how far you travel, only with how long you have been traveling. The key to success in using exercise for weight loss is time—the amount of time you spend exercising. Whether your exercise is nonaerobic or aerobic (see pages 142–45), the more time spent, the greater the benefit in burning calories directly, in raising your RMR, and in fringe benefits such as improved musculoskeletal flexibility and physical and mental relaxation.

Analyzing your exercise achievements in terms of miles rather than minutes may place a destructive focus on speed. Such a focus may cause frustration when you reach your maximum speed in pace walking, for example, and discover (like many of us) that you're not as fast as some other people. Focusing on speed can also lead to injury if you try to reach your maximum before you are physically capable. The exerciser who continues his or her program is the exerciser who exercises at a comfortable pace. Ignore the No Pain, No Gain nonsense. Your gain is the fact you will still be on your program long after the zealots have been forced off theirs by injury, heartbreak, or both.

If you have decided to exercise aerobically (see pages 142–45), your goal should be to work at the level and speed necessary to boost your heart rate over the aerobic minimum. How that compares to anyone else's speed or absolute standard is unimportant. If someone asks you how many miles you run or walk during your workouts, you can state your reply in minutes.

Measuring your workouts in minutes not miles also has practical advantages. If you exercise outdoors, you don't have to measure or plan specific courses. You will probably find one or more favorite routes that you will use over and over again, but your choice will be made solely for pleasure, not necessity. With the minutes approach, the 30-minute outdoor workout simply requires that you pace walk or jog or cycle in one direction for 15 minutes and back for 15 minutes. You're not stuck with the same boring route every day.

Uptown one day, downtown another, through the park a third. You live in the suburbs? Toward your town one day, toward a neighboring town the next, into the country another. All you have to remember is to start home after 15 minutes. Do you prefer mall walking? The same time principle applies. You have the freedom to set your pace according to how you feel and what the weather conditions dictate. You may feel very energetic and want to walk quickly. It may be beastly hot and you may have to walk slowly. Whether going fast or slow, you will spend the same amount of time working out.

GET SET

Keeping an Exercise Log

Just as you maintain a Take Control Eating Log, you should keep a Take Control Exercise Log. In fact, it might provide good cross motivation to maintain the logs together in the same book. In your exercise log you can include scheduled minutes for the day, how many minutes you completed each day, weekly totals, how the workouts went, comments on the weather, thoughts on equipment and clothing, as well as personal notes.

Before You Exercise

Before you start your workout, it's very helpful to take 5 to 10 minutes to warm up. During the warm-up, you first increase the blood circulation to your muscles, then you stretch your muscles to prepare them for strenuous activity. Supple, well-stretched muscles don't directly benefit your heart or lungs, but they will make you much less susceptible to injury.

You should warm up slightly before stretching, because warmer muscles can be stretched more easily without risk of pulls or tears. Start by jogging in place, riding a stationary bicycle at a moderate pace, or doing some calisthenic exercises for two to three minutes. After you get your blood circulating and your muscles warm, stop and stretch.

You should do slow, static stretches, holding a muscle in a stretched-out position for 10 to 30 seconds. As you stretch a muscle, you'll feel a resistance like the tension in a rubber band. Stretch until you feel a slight pull, but *never* to the point of pain. Don't bounce. Bouncing can cause muscle tears. Breathe slowly and steadily; inhale through your nose, exhale through your mouth.

You can become more flexible by stretching, but don't compare yourself with anyone else. Some people are born more flexible than others. Women tend to be more supple than men, and after age 30 both men and women tend to lose flexibility. After several weeks of consistent stretching, your muscle elasticity will increase and you'll be able to stretch further.

After your workout, always give your body a chance to recover slowly and cool down. If you exercise hard and then stop suddenly, your heart continues to pump hard, but your leg muscles no longer help to force the blood back to the heart. If this happens, your blood can "pool" in your lower extremities, leaving your internal organs and brain temporarily short of adequate blood supply. This can cause dizziness, fainting, or vomiting. The cool-down period also helps prevent the buildup of lactic acid, a chemical by-product of exercise. Lactic acid in the muscle leads to muscle soreness. The more you stretch during cool-down, the less likely you are to feel the effects of exercise the next day.

To cool down, continue the activity you've been doing, but at a slower pace, for two or three minutes. If you were jogging, slow down and walk for a few minutes. If you were cycling, pedal in a lower gear. To maintain flexibility, your cool-down should also include at least five minutes of additional stretching *after* you exercise.

The following exercises can be used for both warm-up and cool-down stretching. You may not be able to perform all of them comfortably, at least in the beginning. Remember that "gradual change leads to permanent changes" applies to stretching as well as to other parts of your exercise program. When you first start, just do what works best for you. You can expand your stretching repertory in the weeks and months to come.

Stretching Exercises

Neck stretch. Stand tall with your back straight, and relax your shoulders. Tilt your head to the right, to the rear, to the left, and then forward. Hold each position 10 seconds, repeat 5 to 10 times in each direction. Do not roll your neck, but gently stretch it in each direction.

Shoulder stretch. Stand tall, with your shoulders relaxed. Stretch your arms behind your back and clasp your hands. Lift your arms behind you until you feel a stretch in your arms, chest, and shoulders. Keep your shoulders down and as relaxed as possible. Hold one time for 30 seconds.

Triceps stretch. Reach your left arm overhead and extend your arm behind you as if to scratch your shoulder blade. Place your right hand on your left elbow and gently pull behind you to extend the stretch. Hold one time for 30 seconds. Repeat with your arms switched.

Groin stretch. Sit on the floor, with the soles of your feet pressed together. Hold your ankles and gently press your knees down with your elbows. Keep your back straight. Remember to breathe slowly and steadily. Don't bounce. Hold one time for 30 seconds.

Buttocks stretch. Sit on the floor, with your right leg straight in front of you and your left leg crossed in your lap. Cradle your left ankle and knee in your arms, and gently pull your leg toward your chest. Keep your back straight and your right leg flat on the floor, toes pointed toward the ceiling. Hold one time for 30 seconds. Repeat with the opposite leg.

Hamstring stretch. Sit on the floor with your left leg straight out in front of you and your right leg tucked against your right thigh, close to the body. Reach for the ankle of the extended leg. Flex from the hips and keep your back straight. Don't bounce. You should feel a gentle stretch along your hamstrings, the muscles in the backs of your thighs. Hold one time for 30 seconds, then repeat with the opposite leg.

Modified hamstring stretch. Stand with your left leg resting on the back of a chair or on a counter. Keep your right leg slightly bent. Reach for the ankle of the extended leg. Flex from the hips and keep your back straight. *Don't bounce.* You should feel a gentle stretch along your hamstrings. Hold one time for 30 seconds, then repeat with the opposite leg.

Full-body stretch. Lie flat on your back on the floor, with your arms extended over your head. Stretch your arms and legs, lengthening your arms, shoulders, rib cage, abdominals, spine, legs, and feet. Breathe slowly and steadily. Hold one time for 30 seconds.

Modified quadriceps stretch. (For older individuals or people with back problems. Note: This is not actually a stretch, but a mild contraction, or lengthening of the muscle fibers. It warms up the muscle and may improve flexibility.) Stand tall and hold a chairback or counter to help you keep your balance. Slowly bend your knees. Keep your back straight and your weight over your pelvis. You should feel your quadriceps working—the muscles along the fronts of your thighs. Hold one time for 30 seconds.

Calf stretch. Stand about 2 feet from a wall. Bend your left knee and stretch your right leg behind you. Keep your right leg straight, with your foot flat on the floor and your toes pointed straight ahead. Keep your back straight

TABLE 8.1 *Take Control Exercise Plan*
         Phase I Introductory Program

Week	Mon.	Tues.	Wed.	Thurs.	Fri.	Sat.	Sun.	Total	Comments
				(Times in minutes)					
1	Off	10	Off	10	Off	Off	10	30	Ordinary walking
2	Off	10	Off	10	Off	Off	10	30	
3	Off	20	Off	20	Off	Off	20	60	
4	Off	20	Off	20	Off	Off	20	60	
5	Off	20	Off	20	Off	Off	20	60	Fast walking
6	Off	20	Off	20	Off	Off	20	60	
7	Off	20	Off	20	Off	Off	30	70	
8	Off	20	Off	20	Off	Off	30	70	
9	Off	20	Off	20	Off	Off	20	60	Pace walking
10	Off	20	Off	20	Off	Off	30	70	
11	Off	20	Off	30	Off	Off	30	80	
12	Off	20	Off	30	Off	Off	30	80	
13	Off	30	Off	30	Off	Off	30	90	

and aligned with the extended leg. Lean forward to feel a stretch along your calf muscle. Hold one time for 30 seconds. Repeat with the opposite leg.

To isolate and stretch your ankle, keep your heel flat on the floor and slightly flex the knee of the extended leg. Hold one time for 30 seconds, and repeat with the opposite leg.

Going Through the Plan

The three phases—introduction, development, and maintenance—connect with each other in a logical manner. If you've never exercised, or haven't exercised in a long time, you should begin with Phase I. The tables that follow should be used as guides in deciding how many minutes you will devote to each workout. You can make changes to suit your own needs and schedule, as long as the end results incorporate the Take Control exercise principles.

Phase I is designed to provide a slow and easy introduction to regular exercise. The schedule in Table 8.1 covers a 13-week period and should give you an idea of how you might plan your Introductory Program. However, you can certainly accelerate your movement through it if you progress more rapidly than the program suggests. Some people become enthusiastic early during the program and move ahead quickly, adding minutes and workouts, skipping the early weeks of ordinary walking, and proceeding directly to fast walking or pace walking. If you have recent exercise experience, you may even decide to skip Phase I entirely. But be careful that you don't threaten your long-range goals in your haste to begin a regimen for which you believe you are prepared. If you decide you have gone too far ahead, don't let pride keep you from returning to a more manageable place and pace.

The same general principles should guide you as you go through the Developmental and Maintenance Programs. For example, if you are on Maintenance in Phase III, don't exercise two hours a week by taking one long pace walk each Sunday. However, you need not be a slave to your program, or you will soon want to escape it. If you miss an occasional session, don't feel compelled to make up the lost minutes. But if you feel you would like to catch up, spread the minutes out over several workouts. Also, it will not hurt to do two workouts in a row during the week. If bad weather or travel or an early-morning meeting causes you to miss Tuesday, for example, you can complete that workout on Wednesday and still work out on Thursday as well. It also won't hurt to complete your workouts at different times on different days. If you usually work out in the morning, but on a particular day find it more convenient to work out in the evening, do it.

GO

Phase I: The Introductory Program

Exercise Goals

1. To get in the habit of being a regular exerciser, to make regular exercise a part of your life.
2. To familiarize yourself with the sport(s) or activity that you might like to include in your exercise plan.
3. To get up and over the aerobic minimum time level, 20 minutes, three times each week (if you are aiming to become an aerobic exerciser).

Doing It

The Phase I Introductory Program (see Table 8.1) starts with 30 minutes each week and finishes with 90. If you've never exercised on a regular basis, or haven't done so for a long time, it is suggested you begin here. This program is designed to ease you into a regular schedule of workouts gradually, to help you limber up slowly without causing pain or injury. Because walking is ideal for starting the Take Control Exercise Plan, the table is set up to show a progression from regular walking to fast walking through pace walking. But, as mentioned previously, the plan will work with almost any sport or other physical activity you choose, provided you plan ahead for a graduation to a second and third level of the activity.

Following the example of Table 8.1, take a 10-minute walk, three times each week for the first two weeks. Don't worry about speed or heart rate. Walk at a comfortable pace for a target 10 minutes. You can certainly walk more on days you feel like it. But do not pressure yourself to do so. At this point you have no intermediate objective other than to become a regular exerciser, establish your exercise schedule on your calendar, and make time for it, even if it means getting up earlier in the morning.

During these first two weeks, you have an opportunity to gain control and stay in control. You can enjoy a certain immediate gratification that should help propel you forward. No, you won't lose 20 pounds in two weeks on this plan; it's not that kind of gratification. We're talking about gratification of the mind that often accompanies the knowledge that you can take control of your life and make positive changes.

In the first two weeks, you can take a big step toward making regular exercise a permanent part of your life. In these two weeks you can confirm that you are ready to take responsibility for how you look and how you feel about yourself.

During the second two weeks, walk at a comfortable pace for 20 minutes continuing your loosening-up process, becoming accustomed to being on a workout schedule, while doubling the time that you spend on each one. As your workouts increase in length, you can explore different routes.

In weeks five through eight, continue to walk, but pick up the pace. We are not talking about pace walking. Don't worry about armswing, just try for smoothness and comfort, while walking faster than an amble. At this point you don't want to burden yourself with walking technique, but you can work on developing a steady, smooth, easy rhythm to your walking. You might be listening to music on your portable headset or imagining a piece of music to which you can step along. On a practical level, rhythmic walking exercises more of your body's muscles, makes walking less tiring, and prepares you for pace walking.

In week nine, you pace walk. Don't worry about all the technical details.

Focus on four points: (1) relaxed upper body, no scrunched shoulders; (2) strong armswing; (3) firm heelstrike, rolling forward over the sole of your walking shoe to a lifting push-off from your toes; (4) smooth, steady rhythm: rockin', rollin', and liftin'. You will soon become more comfortable with the gait. Don't worry about how fast you're walking; focus on incorporating regular exercise into your life-style.

Aerobic Exercise

We noted in chapter 7 that you do not have to exercise aerobically in order to lose weight. Aerobic exercise primarily benefits your cardiovascular system. However, if you work up to aerobic exercise, you will be using your weight-loss workout time more efficiently. Aerobic exercise leads to both improved health and improved fitness. Three hours of aerobic exercise each week is all you need on a long-term basis to attain maximum health benefits from your efforts. However, fitness continues to improve if you work out up to a total of 10 to 12 hours each week. Improved fitness is of course required for many physical activities, such as long-distance racing, but you do not need more than three hours of aerobic exercise each week for health benefits. None of the programs described in this book requires more than three hours a week, except the Maintenance Double Plus in Phase III.

Aerobic Exercise and Your Heart Rate

Aerobic exercise means using large muscle groups (e.g., arms and shoulders, buttocks and legs) to increase muscle oxygen uptake above a certain level. But we can't walk around with meters that measure muscle oxygen uptake. For the healthy person without heart disease, nature provides a good measurement of muscle oxygen uptake that is simple for anyone to take. It is the heart rate. Exercise physiology has determined that when your heart rate rises above a certain level, you are doing aerobic exercise.

There is a simple, standard formula for finding your aerobic heart rate level. More sophisticated formulae are available for the well-trained athlete. But for our purposes, the following calculation is adequate. First, subtract your age from the number 220. Exercise physiologists call the remainder the *theoretical maximum heart rate*. It is called a *theoretical* maximum because your true maximum, the rate above which your heart simply cannot beat, is not always precisely the same in every person of the same age. But among most healthy people, the true maximum is close to the theoretical maximum.

Second, take 60 percent of the number that expresses your theoretical

TABLE 8.2 *Minimum Aerobic Heart Rates for Selected Ages*
(60 percent of theoretical maximum heart rate)

Age	Heart Rate	Age	Heart Rate
21	119	55	99
25	117	60	96
30	114	65	93
35	111	70	90
39	109	75	87
40	108	80	84
45	105	85	81
50	102	90	78

maximum heart rate. The result is the minimum *target heart rate* (THR) that you need to achieve to be sure that the exercise you are doing is aerobic. Table 8.2 shows the THR for some sample ages. To be on the safe side, you should never exercise so strenuously that your heart rate rises above 80 percent of your theoretical maximum. So, for safe aerobic exercise, try to get your heart beating within its optimum range. That's 220 minus your age multiplied by .8 for the upper limit; multiplied by .6 for the lower limit.

How to determine your heart rate. You will need either a digital watch with a seconds readout or a regular watch with a second hand. Out on the road, in the pool, or on your stationary bike, you will find it much easier to take your pulse at the carotid artery than at the wrist. On the side of your neck is a thick band of muscle that runs from the angle at the back of the lower jaw to the notch that marks the middle of the collarbone. Use the index and middle fingers of one hand to feel along the front border of the muscle band on the opposite side (e.g., use the right hand to feel the left side of the neck). About halfway down you will feel a large pulsating blood vessel, the carotid artery—the main vessel on each side that provides blood to the brain. You should be able to find it fairly easily; if not, try using the other hand.

You may also take the pulse in your wrist. If you are wearing your watch on your right wrist, turn your left hand palm up. Place the index and second fingers of your right hand just above your left wrist at the thumb side. You should feel a depression at this point. Gently press your fingers into that depression until you can feel the pulse and count beats from one 10-second break on your watch to the next. Because 10 seconds represent only one-sixth of a minute, you will have to multiply your number by 6 to obtain your heart rate, measured always in beats per minute.

Caution: Do not attempt to take the carotid pulse on both sides of your neck simultaneously. Doing so could cause you to faint, or worse. **Taking it on one side at a time is perfectly safe, unless you have hardening of the arteries (arteriosclerosis) in one or both of your carotid arteries. If you have any suspicion that you might have carotid artery disease, check with your physician before taking your pulse in this manner.**

If you're using a digital watch it may be easier to count beats within a 6-second interval and then multiply by 10. You may think that such a method cannot be that accurate, for only by coincidence will a last full beat fall conveniently within the time interval. If you want to measure it more accurately, counting for 15 seconds and multiplying by 4 somewhat solves the problem, because the extra beat you've included counts for only 4, not 6 or 10.

The longer you count, the more accurate your measurements. But remember that if you have been exercising strenuously and stop to read your pulse, your heart rate is slowing as you count beats. Thus, if you count beats for a minute, you will get a reading of the average rate as your heart rate slowed through the minute.

But the purpose of taking your pulse is not to find a precise number. A rough count will indicate if you are exercising intensively enough so that your heart rate is up in the aerobic range, and yet not so strenuously that you're exceeding your maximum safe rate.

The Standards for Aerobic Exercise

If you want to become aerobically fit as well as lose weight, you should aim to reach the following standards, established by the American College of Sports Medicine:

- Exercise three to five days each week.
- Warm up for 5 to 10 minutes before each aerobic activity session.
- Maintain your desired exercise intensity for 20 to 60 minutes.

• Gradually decrease your activity to cool down, and stretch for 5 to 10 minutes.

Whether or not you have decided to become an aerobic exerciser, it is probably a good idea, starting in week five, to take your pulse halfway through and at the end of each workout. You may find that it's in the aerobic range. If this is not the case, don't worry about it. You don't have to be in the aerobic range to reach your goals. If you have decided to work up to aerobic exercise eventually, then as you speed your pace, and especially as you accentuate and strengthen your armswing in pace walking, your heart rate will rise.

Remember: If you are a beginning exerciser, and your heart rate rises above 65 percent of your theoretical maximum, it is too high. You're going too fast. Slow down and maintain a slower pace for another week before increasing your speed. If, and only if, you are going to be an aerobic exerciser, 65 to 70 percent of your theoretical maximum is a good rate to aim for in any sport you use in the Take Control plan.

If during exercise or shortly thereafter you experience palpitations, chest pressure, or pain radiating to your neck, arms, or back, go to the nearest hospital emergency room at once.

Intermediate Outcomes

Before the end of the first 13 weeks, almost everyone will see and feel results. Since you are combining the Take Control Eating Plan with the Take Control Exercise Plan, you will have lost some weight and fat. For example, a woman of average height who is 25 or more pounds above her desired weight may lose 10 to 15 pounds in the first 13 weeks, about a pound a week on average. (Fewer pounds are lost during the beginning weeks of this program than at the end.) That weight loss may not seem like a lot, but if you follow the Take Control advice on eating and exercise, those pounds will stay off, unlike many of the pounds you lost and regained on fad diets.

However, if you don't lose as much as 15 or 20 pounds in the first 13 weeks, don't worry about it. Your body probably needs more time to adapt its metabolism and change the way it uses energy. You should continue to exercise regularly, perhaps somewhat more vigorously, to help raise your RMR sufficiently to use the extra calories you have stored as fat.

Even if you don't lose much weight, if you exercise regularly, even if modestly, you will most likely lose fat and add muscle. The failure of your bathroom scale to reflect your progress is related to the fact that muscle is heavier than fat. You can find satisfaction in knowing you have probably redistributed a few of your pounds.

As you continue to exercise, building muscle, and losing fat, your weight may not constantly decline. In fact, as you add muscle mass, you may gain a few pounds. People who haven't seen you in a while may say, "You've really lost weight," when you have actually only substituted muscle for fat. In any case, you will probably look better and feel both healthier and better about yourself.

Roadblocks You May Encounter and How to Overcome Them

You may encounter a series of roadblocks on the way to becoming a regular exerciser. The most important thing to remember is that you are not alone. Most people who are now regular exercisers have met these roadblocks, and most have dealt with them successfully. Here are some tips to help you do the same.

1. "I don't like this." First, isolate what it is you don't like. If it's the regular aspect of exercising, the only solution is to limit the amount of time: Lower the number of minutes and confine your walking to short sessions, but continue to try to build those sessions into your routine. Do not try to exercise more than three times a week, if you are thinking that your dislike stems from the number of times you have to go out.

Second, find a fantasy of success or achievement on which you can concentrate while exercising, each episode of the fantasy to be continued during your next session. You can almost live another life while you exercise.

Third, if you don't like the activity you have chosen, try another one. And if that doesn't work, choose a third. The range of suitable sports/activities is very broad (see chapter 9).

2. "It hurts." Again, the first thing to do is to determine what hurts. Did you injure yourself? Injury is indicated by pain that doesn't go away, redness, swelling, and limitation of motion in the affected area. If this happens, stop and see a physician.

However, if the pain is a result of stiffness from long disuse, the only way to treat that kind of pain is to stop for a period of time, not something you want to do at the beginning of your program. So, *prevention* is the key word here.

Take it easy in the beginning. Go slowly and do not exercise too long during each session.

Second, you may have a problem with your equipment, especially your shoes. A pair of shoes that does not fit can cause many problems—from heel and toe blisters to shin splints—that can make continuing to exercise extremely uncomfortable, if not impossible. It is understandable that you don't want to spend a lot of money for a good pair of walking or aerobic shoes until you are truly committed to an exercise program, but if you have nothing to wear except an old pair of sneakers, you may have to invest in a pair of quality walking shoes.

Deciding you may quit, and thus may as well use bad shoes that cause pain, which in turn causes you to quit, represents a classic self-fulfilling prophecy. A comfortable, stylish pair of new shoes may be the investment that keeps you from quitting too easily.

3. "I don't like getting up early in the morning." Remember, at the beginning of your Take Control Exercise Plan, you can put the bulk of your workout minutes into the weekends, although that is not recommended. And you can continue your weekend workouts until you are ready to increase the number of midweek workouts and the time you will devote to each. If you don't like the morning, how about before or after dinner? Within the constraints of consistency and regularity, there is plenty of room for flexibility in the Take Control program.

4. "This is not working." What do you mean by "not working"? You mean that you've been at it almost a month and still don't look like Arnold or Cher? You haven't lost all the weight you wanted to lose in the two months since you've started? Immediate gratification continues to elude you?

Review the material in the earlier chapters on metabolism, goal setting, and how the drive for immediate gratification may actually hinder your goal of achieving permanent weight loss. Be happy you have started your program, that you are maintaining your plan, and that whether or not you are losing weight you are becoming healthier and stronger, even if only imperceptibly at this point.

If you are not yet in good physical condition after a month or two, and you attribute that to the program "not working," please understand that you are starting from the beginning. If you are following the recommended gradual, one-step-at-a-time approach, and if you are like most people, you may well not feel that you are in shape for at least four months, maybe six. This program takes time. But the trade-off is that if you do it this way, you are more likely to continue the program indefinitely, until it becomes as much a part of your routine as showering and brushing your teeth.

Making Exercise a Part of Your Daily Routines

One way to help you obtain your exercise goals is to include exercise in the routines of your daily life. Try one or more of the following:

- Get off the subway one stop, or the bus five stops, from your destination and walk the rest of the way.
- If you live within a mile or two of work or school, walk there instead of driving or using public transportation.
- If you must drive, park at the far end of the lot, or even at another lot a half-mile from your destination.
- Walk to the supermarket for food shopping, and take the food home the old-fashioned way, in a shopping cart or a wagon.
- Walk to the mall. If it is too far from your home to walk, park in the mall lot as far away from the buildings as possible. Walk through the mall, rather than drive from store to store.
- You certainly know this one: Whenever possible, use the stairs instead of the elevator.

At the end of the first 13 weeks, you should be ready to move on to Phase II.

Phase II: The Developmental Program

Exercise Goals

1. To firmly establish regular exercise as part of your life.
2. To work up to the "aerobic max" of three hours a week of regular exercise (if it's one of your objectives).

Phase II (Table 8.3) has four workouts each week, starting in week three of your program. Two are on weekdays, and two are on weekend days. This phase demands more time than Phase I. Yet in each week, one-half or more of the total minutes are on the two weekend days. This makes life easier for the Take Control exerciser who works outside the home. Certainly, if you work outside the home on weekends and are off during the week, you can rearrange these schedules to meet your own needs.

This phase of your program increases your regular exercise to two or three hours a week. At the end of Phase II, you will have been on an exercise schedule

TABLE 8.3 *Take Control Exercise Plan*
         Phase II   Developmental Program

Week	Mon.	Tues.	Wed.	Thurs.	Fri.	Sat.	Sun.	Total
			(Times in minutes)					
1	Off	Off	Off	Off	Off	Off	Off	Off
2	Off	20	Off	20	Off	Off	20	60
3	Off	20	Off	20	Off	20	20	80
4	Off	20	Off	20	Off	20	30	90
5	Off	20	Off	30	Off	20	30	100
6	Off	20	Off	30	Off	20	40	110
7	Off	30	Off	30	Off	30	30	120
8	Off	30	Off	30	Off	30	40	130
9	Off	30	Off	40	Off	30	40	140
10	Off	30	Off	40	Off	30	50	150
11	Off	40	Off	30	Off	30	60	160
12	Off	40	Off	30	Off	40	60	170
13	Off	30	Off	40	Off	50	60	180

for 26 weeks. For most people at this stage, exercise is a regular part of their lives and they should be able to continue exercising indefinitely.

According to Take Control principles, rest should be scheduled regularly. Phase II begins with a week off. In Phase III time off is scheduled regularly every 13 weeks. This rests your mind and body. Don't worry about losing your conditioning. Your developing physical shape will not revert to its pre–Take Control form in a week, as long as you continue your Take Control Eating Plan. By taking a week off in the exercise program you help prevent exercise burnout.

After the week off, there is a light week with total time well below the last week of the Introductory Program. After that, the weekly time requirement begins to build again, as it does steadily throughout the program. Notice how the workout lengths vary within each week, following the Bowerman hard-easy principle.

The Developmental Program maxes out at three hours. Virtually anyone can reach that level safely and comfortably. However, if you know in advance that in Phase III you are going to use Maintenance rather than one of the other programs, go only through week 9 of Phase II and then repeat weeks 6 through 9 again, substituting them for weeks 10 through 13.

In either case, you will be using the latter part of Phase II to perfect your technique and enhance your endurance. You will be in better shape than before. If you are exercising aerobically, you will probably find that in order to boost your heart rate above the aerobic minimum you will have to work much harder than you did at the beginning of the program. In pace walking, you will understand the importance of armswing.

When you complete the Developmental Program, you have become a regular exerciser. Congratulate yourself. You may have learned a new sport, or at least have become one of the best on your block at whatever activity you have chosen as your exercise. You are becoming healthier. If you have chosen aerobics, your heart and lungs are more fit than they've been since you were young. Your stamina and endurance have increased markedly. You may discover you have a special talent in the sport you have chosen, opening a whole new vista for you. You will continue to lose weight and by losing fat, redistribute some of your remaining weight.

Reward yourself. Go out and buy that great sports outfit you have been wanting. Get away for a special weekend, with or without exercise as a part of it. Or—dare I say it?—have that double hot-fudge sundae that you have been refusing for the last three months.

Phase III: The Maintenance Program

Exercise Goals

1. To confirm your commitment to regular exercise.
2. To settle upon the maintenance program that is best for you.
3. To become comfortable with and skilled in the sport(s) you have selected for your Take Control Exercise Plan.

Phase III gives you three choices: Maintenance, Maintenance Plus, and Maintenance Double Plus. In Maintenance you work out every other day—three days one week, four the next. Your total time is two hours a week. Maintenance Plus gives you four workouts a week, for a total of three hours. Maintenance Double Plus gives you five workouts a week for a total of four hours. If you begin to feel like going beyond four hours a week, you're ready for a racing program; even if you're not going to race, see Appendix C. If you are interested in setting up noncompetitive races for pace walkers, see Appendix D. You also have the option of changing maintenance programs from quarter to quarter of the year.

Maintenance. In this program (Table 8.4), you again start with a week off.

TABLE 8.4 *Take Control Exercise Plan*
          Phase III   Maintenance Program

Week	Mon.	Tues.	Wed.	Thurs.	Fri.	Sat.	Sun.	Total
				(Times in minutes)				
1	Off	Off	Off	Off	Off	Off	Off	Off
2	Off	30	Off	30	Off	Off	40	100
3	30	Off	40	Off	20	Off	40	130
4	Off	40	Off	30	Off	40	Off	110
5	30	Off	40	Off	20	Off	40	130
6	Off	40	Off	30	Off	60	Off	130
7	20	Off	30	Off	30	Off	40	120
8	Off	40	Off	30	Off	50	Off	120
9	20	Off	40	Off	20	Off	60	140
10	Off	30	Off	30	Off	40	Off	100
11	20	Off	30	Off	20	Off	40	110
12	Off	40	Off	30	Off	60	Off	130
13	20	Off	30	Off	30	Off	40	120

Rest, relax, feel good about yourself. Over the remaining 12 weeks of this program you will average two hours of exercise each week. This is the weekly time equivalent for the majority of regular runners in the United States. It is about double the American College of Sports Medicine's minimum recommended time for aerobic health and fitness (20 minutes, three times a week). Very few people who exercise regularly actually do only the minimum. Most people who become physically active for health reasons seem naturally compelled to do more. Thus, you may find two hours a week comfortable and productive.

The every-other-day schedule of the Maintenance Program has been standard among weight lifters for years. Muscle fibers that have been worked hard generally take about 48 hours to recover. Since there is only one weekend day per week in this program, it is impossible to concentrate the workout minutes on the weekends. But the program is balanced. There is no weekday workout of more than 40 minutes, with the average being about 30. Again you will notice the gradual variation in both session length and minutes per week over time.

Maintenance Plus. The Maintenance Plus Program (Table 8.5) provides an average of three hours of aerobic exercise a week for the 12 weeks of the program that follow the obligatory first week off. You can begin Maintenance

TABLE 8.5 *Take Control Exercise Plan*
           Phase III   Maintenance Plus Program

Week	Mon.	Tues.	Wed.	Thurs.	Fri.	Sat.	Sun.	Total
				(Times in minutes)				
1	Off	Off	Off	Off	Off	Off	Off	Off
2	Off	30	Off	40	Off	30	50	150
3	Off	30	Off	50	Off	40	60	180
4	Off	40	Off	40	Off	50	80	210
5	Off	30	Off	50	Off	40	60	180
6	Off	50	Off	30	Off	50	70	200
7	Off	40	Off	30	Off	30	60	180
8	Off	30	Off	50	Off	40	60	180
9	Off	30	Off	40	Off	30	50	150
10	Off	30	Off	50	Off	40	50	170
11	Off	40	Off	30	Off	50	70	190
12	Off	40	Off	40	Off	50	80	210
13	Off	30	Off	50	Off	40	60	180

Plus immediately after Phase II. More than half the total minutes are concentrated in the two weekend days. If done aerobically, Maintenance Plus requires a three-hour maximum for health benefits. Many Take Control exercisers will find this to be a very comfortable permanent program.

Maintenance Double Plus. The Maintenance Double Plus Program (Table 8.6) provides an average of four hours each week, spread over five workouts. If one hour is a comfortable workout time for you, you can modify this program to do the four hours in four workouts. Otherwise, take one of the five sessions in Maintenance Double Plus, divide by four, and add the minutes to each of the remaining four workouts.

This program is the equivalent of about 20 to 25 miles of fast pace walking or running a week. If you like this program, you have probably fallen in love with regular exercise. You may also like sport for its own sake, not just what it does for your mind and body. At this point you may be ready to try doing two or more sports in the same program. If so, pace training should appeal to you.

TABLE 8.6 *Take Control Exercise Plan*
Phase III   Maintenance Double Plus Program

Week	Mon.	Tues.	Wed.	Thurs.	Fri.	Sat.	Sun.	Total
				(Times in minutes)				
1	Off	Off	Off	Off	Off	Off	Off	Off
2	Off	30	40	Off	30	40	70	210
3	Off	30	50	Off	40	50	70	240
4	Off	40	40	Off	50	60	80	270
5	Off	30	50	Off	30	50	80	240
6	Off	50	30	Off	30	60	90	260
7	Off	40	30	Off	30	50	70	220
8	Off	30	50	Off	30	60	70	240
9	Off	30	40	Off	30	50	60	210
10	Off	30	50	Off	30	60	70	230
11	Off	40	30	Off	40	60	80	250
12	Off	40	40	Off	40	60	90	270
13	Off	30	50	Off	30	70	60	240

Pace Training

Pace training is working out in two or more sports in the same program, for health, fitness, or fun. It is a form of cross training, used by single-sport racers who want to achieve and maintain a high level of aerobic fitness while diminishing their risk of overuse injury. We use the term *cross training* when talking about racers, and *pace training* when talking about regular exercisers. Pace training focuses on enjoyment of sport in general, not on skill or speed in any one sport in particular.

Pace training recognizes that any aerobic exercise improves the fitness level of the heart. Your heart can't tell the difference between pace walking, rowing, or aerobic dancing. It only knows that it is being required to pump more oxygen-rich blood to distant muscles. Cumulatively, your aerobic fitness will improve regardless of how many aerobic sports you put together in your particular program.

In pace training you choose two or more sports in which you wish to participate. You will probably be on the Maintenance Double Plus Program. You might, for example, pace walk on two of the five workout days each week, swim once, and cycle indoors twice. You can mix and match the sports as you please.

Pace training is designed to be fun and reduce injury risk, but it is not magic and it is not painless. As you know by now, there are no magical solutions for becoming healthy and fit through exercise. Pace training requires commitment, as do all of the Take Control phases. It requires mental discipline, consistency, and regularity. But it can make your Take Control Exercise Plan more fun and beneficial for you.

Major Advantages of Pace Training

Pace training has five major advantages over single-sport training:

1. You significantly reduce the boredom potential of regular exercise by building psychological and physical variety into your training program.
2. You exercise and develop two or more major muscle groups at the same time, and promote muscle balance.
3. Engaging in two activities reduces the risk of both intrinsic and extrinsic injury, because demands are made on a second group of muscles instead of overburdening a single group.
4. If you work out aerobically, you build up your cardiovascular fitness without risking strain or overuse of any single major muscle group.
5. If you work out aerobically, you improve the ability of all the muscles in your body to use the oxygen supplied to them by the blood.

Each major health and fitness sport focuses on particular groups of muscles. Running mainly involves the calf muscles and the hamstrings (those at the backs of the thighs), while also working the fronts of the thighs (quadriceps, or "quads") and the lower back. Pace walking uses leg muscles, but also exercises hip and lower back muscles. In addition, by using a vigorous armswing, it exercises the muscles of the upper back and shoulders. Bicycling focuses on the quads and lower back muscles; if cleats are used and a pull-up is incorporated into the pedal stroke (see chapter 9), focus is placed on the calves. Free-style swimming is primarily an upper body sport.

If you are going to concentrate on only one of the major workout sports for your Take Control Exercise Plan, only pace walking, weight training, or aerobic dance (and its variants) will provide a relatively complete body workout. If you choose it, pace training provides training for whole parts of the body by exercising the separate major muscle groups in separate sports.

Knowing When to Slow Down

As you begin your Take Control Exercise Plan, you know you will need mental discipline, but you should be aware that the discipline is of two kinds. First, you will need discipline to stay with your program, to make regular exercise a part of your life, to recognize its intrusiveness and accept and adapt to it. Second, you will need mental discipline to avoid trying to do too much, to learn what some athletes call "staying within yourself." In a way this second discipline is related to goal setting. Be clear about your goals, and make sure the goals you decide upon are reasonable. Don't design a program that is more than you can achieve in terms of time and your current athletic ability.

Explore your limits. Most of us never reach them. But also recognize your limitations. Regular exercise is for health, fitness, weight loss, and feeling good. It should not build anxiety, frustration, anger, isolation, and stress. If you have it in you to become a good athlete as well as a regular exerciser, these talents and inclinations will surface.

If necessary, take more time off than suggested in the Take Control plan. It won't hurt you. Some people believe that if you stop exercising aerobically for three or four weeks, you will lose all the conditioning you had developed. Research shows that this is true only for people who haven't been working out for very long. Once you become fit, it would take three to five months of not working out for you to lose entirely the gains you made.

If you are reasonably fit, you can take breaks of two to three weeks without much effect on fitness, provided you are in control of the break. It seems that if you *have* to stop because of injury, you go downhill fairly quickly, both in your fitness level and in your attitude. But apparently, if you decide that you simply *want* to stop for a while, you don't lose much.

On the other hand, an important part of mental discipline for the Take Control exerciser is to be able to distinguish times you need a break from times you have to push yourself. This skill can be developed only through trial and error. You may have trouble getting up in the morning for your workout, but find that once you are up, dressed, and out of the house things go well, both during and after the workout. That happens to regular exercisers all the time. All you needed to do was to push yourself through a mild case of the blahs, exercise the discipline to reject snuggling deeper under the covers.

Knowing When to Stop

Suppose you have decided you want to lose weight and fat and you need to be on Pathway C in order to do that. You begin the Take Control Exercise Plan.

You give it a reasonable and legitimate effort. You try pace walking and some of the other sports; you try them alone and in combinations. Nothing works. You can't get on a regular schedule. And further, you find that you are not getting any of the hoped-for benefits, or, if you are, you feel that the effort is not worth the reward.

You haven't been forced to lose weight. You have the right to stop. And if you do, you shouldn't feel guilty about it. Regular exercise, aerobic or non-aerobic, is good for almost everyone. Maybe it will not work for you at this time. Maybe in six months or a year you'll feel differently. Maybe that inner motivation isn't there yet. Maybe it never will be. That's okay. Neither being overweight nor being sedentary means that you are a bad person.

If you do not like regular exercise and find you are not getting anything out of it, stop. If you try to continue, you will become angry, frustrated, and more at risk for injury. So, you need mental discipline to know when to stop as well as when to continue.

9

Sports Techniques and Equipment

YOU DON'T HAVE to be an expert to benefit fully from any sports or regular exercise activities. A good technique, however, makes whatever sport you are doing more comfortable and enjoyable, and decreases the likelihood of injury. It also gives you that feeling of being in control—so important to success in weight loss.

On the other hand, it's not a good idea to become a technique fanatic. Too much focus on technique, especially if you have trouble learning some of the finer points, can rob you of enjoyment in the sport. So, as always, resist perfectionism. Find the happy medium and stay in control.

Choosing the right equipment (including clothing) is important, too, for many of the same reasons. Good equipment makes the sport or activity more comfortable, more fun, and safer in terms both of intrinsic (overuse) and extrinsic (external causes) injury risk. It's not necessary to spend a lot of money, though. In the beginning, good, moderately priced equipment will do. Later on, if you become seriously interested in a particular activity, you can spend money on top equipment.

Comparison of Calorie Use

Even though we usually refrain from calorie counting in this book, you may want to review the comparison of calories expended per hour among various sports (see Table 9.1). These figures are based on the assumption that the sports are done aerobically, and that average speeds are maintained. The actual number of calories used will vary among participating individuals.

TABLE 9.1 *Calorie Use for Various Sports*

Activity (Average Intensity)	Calories Burned per Minute at a Weight of					
	120	140	160	180	200	220
Aerobic dance/exercise	5.7	6.6	7.5	8.5	9.4	10.3
Calisthenics, ice/roller skating, soccer, downhill skiing	4.7	5.5	6.3	7.1	7.8	8.6
Jumping rope	9.4	10.9	12.5	14.0	15.6	17.1
Cross-country skiing, swimming	6.6	7.7	8.8	9.8	10.9	12.0
Handball, racketball, squash, tennis (singles)	7.5	8.8	10.0	11.2	12.5	13.7
Walking (4 mph)	4.7	5.5	6.3	7.1	7.8	8.6
Jogging (11 minutes per mile)	8.4	9.8	11.2	12.6	14.0	15.4
Bicycling (13 mph)	9.1	10.5	11.9	13.3	14.7	16.1

Source: American College of Sports Medicine

TECHNIQUE

Walking

Ordinary walking is a simple activity we usually do without thinking about it. You decide to move from point A to point B, and you put one foot in front of the other until you reach point B. Walking is far down the list of efficient transportation methods, but it remains at the top when rated for the health benefits it provides.

Walking in the park or strolling on a Sunday afternoon on the boardwalk while looking out over the water are family, social, or individual activities that can be pursued for their own benefit. Looking at the clouds, foliage, vistas, animals, and other people can be mind expanding, restful, and at the same time invigorating. Ambling at a leisurely pace while conversing with a friend, a child, or other loved one can be an especially enjoyable experience. Many sightseers will tell you that the best way to see any place, whether a large city, small town, or countryside, is to walk through it slowly, experiencing the special sights, sounds, and smells of the place.

Hiking—along country trails, through the mountains, or along the beach—is an enjoyable sport in its own right. It can provide even richer and more varied experiences when combined with activities such as camping or orienteering. Hiking in mountainous terrain can lead to the invigorating and demanding sport of mountain climbing. These forms, variants, and extensions of walking are sports that have been popular for many, many years in many countries.

In the past few years, as part of an increased interest in aerobic exercise in our country, the popularity of fast walking has grown rapidly. Walking has become an accepted aerobic sport, even by such former skeptics as George Sheehan, M.D., generally known as the guru of running for health and fitness. In 1986, after making some earlier disparaging remarks, Dr. Sheehan described walking as "the best exercise of all."

If you haven't been doing any exercising, if you're totally out of shape, just walking at a pace slightly faster than normal will probably raise your heart rate into your aerobic range, whether or not you intend to get it there. You may find that after just a few weeks of walking slightly faster than usual, your heart rate will no longer rise to the aerobic level, and you may have to walk with a determined gait to maintain the sport at an aerobic level. You will now, by definition, be fast walking.

As pointed out previously, regular exercise does not have to be aerobic to be beneficial for weight and fat loss. Any regular exercise will burn excess calories stored in fat and raise the resting metabolic rate. But if the exercise is aerobic, you will burn more calories in the same amount of time, and you will receive the other health benefits of aerobic exercise.

Of course, walking is not the only sport that can be done either aerobically or not. You can run so slowly that your heart rate does not rise above the lower threshold of the aerobic range. A leisurely bike ride around the park at 8 to 10 miles per hour will be an aerobic exercise for some people but not for others. However, most people will have to bike at 13 to 15 miles per hour, a pretty good clip, for the sport to be aerobic. The same applies to cross-country skiing or rowing or swimming or most of the other aerobic sports. To become aerobic, each must be done with a certain degree of intensity, at some speed that will push your heart rate above your threshold for aerobic exercise.

Pace Walking

Pace walking is a special form of ordinary walking: aerobic walking for sport, exercise, and health, at your own pace. Pace walking will do for your body and your mind what any of the other exercises or sports will do when they are done at the same level of intensity for the same amount of time.

Pace walking (also known as health walking, fitness walking, or sports walking) is simple, rhythmic, relatively pain free, and inexpensive. If you're overweight or out of shape, the gentleness and naturalness of pace walking are perfectly suited for you at the beginning of your Take Control Exercise Plan. Further, the excess weight that you have will be an advantage in that it will make the sport aerobic at a relatively low level of exertion, until you lose some of that weight. So, if you don't already have experience in another sport that you are eager to return to, try pace walking to get you started as a regular exerciser.

The Pace-Walking Gait

The basics. Pace walking is simple. You walk fast with a purposeful stride of medium length. With each stride, you land on your heel, roll forward along the outside of your foot, and push off your toes into the next stride. As you push off, you should bend your toes just about as far as they can go. Your back should be comfortably straight but not rigid. Your head should be up, shoulders relaxed and dropped.

In pace walking, unlike running, the arm motion is as important as leg motion. Most people find it impossible to walk fast enough to get the heart rate up into the aerobic range without a determined, rhythmic swing of the arms. With your elbows comfortably bent, the armswing should be forward and back, in the direction you are moving. Try not to move your arms across your chest. While that may look attractive and feel vigorous, it hinders your forward momentum, and may lead to body imbalance and possible injury.

Obviously, your left arm should go forward with your right leg, and vice versa. Your fingers should be slightly cupped, your fists never clenched. As your arm swings forward, your hand should reach about to upper chest level. On each swing back, you should stop when you feel your back shoulder muscles gently but firmly stretching. It is the combination of leg stride and armswing that provides one of the advantages pace walking has over most other major aerobic sports. Unlike swimming, biking, and running, pace walking exercises two—not just one—of the major muscle groups. Although rowing and cross-country skiing also do this, they are limited access/limited participation sports. Of the other major sports, only aerobic dance and its variations consistently work more than one major muscle group.

Some refinements. After you master the basics of stride, posture, and arm-swing, you can refine your technique. For example, point your feet straight ahead, keeping them as close as possible to an imaginary white line along which you walk—not walking on that white line, but straddling it to help keep you balanced and level.

You can rotate your hip forward with the forward motion of the leg on the same side, if you feel comfortable doing it. This will make your gait something like that of race walking. But rotation of the hip is not essential. Most important, be sure that one foot is always on the ground. That's what makes pace walking walking, and a more gentle sport. In running, you are airborne between each step, leading to a foot strike of considerably greater pressure than in walking.

Race walking. A technically demanding sport, race walking requires a different gait from that of pace walking. Race walkers can move remarkably fast, up to 7 minutes a mile for 30 miles (50 kilometers) in a race walking marathon. That's a faster pace than many runners achieve in a 26.2-mile (43.7 kilometers) marathon. Reaching that speed in race walking requires a complex hip rotation that amuses many people. It may look funny, but it is the most efficient way to walk. It lengthens the stride without overstretching the leg, and it permits much higher cadences than the ordinary walker can achieve.

Race walking also has rules. In addition to the general requirement that at least one foot must always be on the ground, the knee of the weight-bearing leg must be straight for at least an instant as the body passes over it. This is difficult to do unless you practice for a while. In race walking competitions there are judges on the course to make sure that competitors follow the rules.

Speed. Speed potential in pace walking is a combination of natural ability, practice, and level of fitness. In the beginning, you will probably walk at a pace of 15 to 18 minutes a mile. As a basis for comparison, normal walking covers a mile in about 20 minutes. With some practice you will find yourself walking 13 to 14 minutes a mile; 11 to 12 minutes a mile is an excellent speed in pace walking. If you want to walk faster than that, you will probably have to learn to race walk.

Balance, smoothness, rhythm, and lift. Very important to an effective, comfortable, efficient pace walking gait are balance, smoothness, rhythm, and lift. You should strive for as little extraneous body motion as possible. If you watch some race walkers, you will notice hardly any up-and-down movement to their heads. Why is that important? Because in walking, we want to move forward, not up and down, or side to side. Your head and torso should be motionless. Following through all the way on each step is a key to fluidity of motion—another goal of pace walking. Consistent technique in follow-through, lift, and rhythm—each contributes to the other—helps make pace walking fun.

Other Considerations of Pace Walking

Breathing. You will find it helpful if your breathing is as rhythmic as your gait. When you begin ordinary walking in the Take Control Exercise Plan, you will probably not be breathing too hard. But as your proficiency and stamina increase, you will be able to go faster; both your rate and depth of breathing will rise. Deep breathing is important. With each breath, you will be bringing in more oxygen and expelling more carbon dioxide. Using your diaphragm to expand your lungs downward and using your chest muscles to expand the rib cage outward will help you breathe as deeply as possible. As your walking speed and breathing rate pick up, you may find that timing your breathing to your steps makes maintaining your rhythm easier and more comfortable. For example, you might breathe in for three paces, out for three paces.

Posture. You should be relaxed. While standing straight, you should not be rigidly upright. Tense muscles lead to strain and pain. Also, you want your upper body nice and loose so that you can develop a smooth, rhythmic, full armswing. As your speed increases, you may be more comfortable if you bend forward slightly. Make sure you are bending from the hips, not at the waist. If you bend at the waist you will inhibit the full movement of your diaphragm, and interfere with your breathing.

Stride length. Stride length varies from person to person; it may also change during workouts. You will probably take short steps going uphill, long ones going downhill. When you are on level ground, the shorter you make your stride, the faster you can move your legs. An aerobic heart rate can be produced either way, with short, quick strides or with long, easier ones.

Be sure not to overstride, or take steps that require you to reach too far forward with your foot. This will only lead to imbalance and possible injury. Since your Take Control workouts are measured in minutes, not miles, you don't have to worry about covering huge tracts of ground. Taking longer steps will not get you through your workout any more quickly. Nor will shorter steps mean a longer workout. Above all, your stride length should be one that is most comfortable for you.

Pace walking with weights. Pace walking with weights can add to the vigor of your workout and help raise your heart rate into your aerobic range without requiring you to increase your speed. This is especially helpful for people who are already in reasonably good aerobic shape and would otherwise have to push their pace to raise their heart rate above the aerobic minimum.

Pace walking with weights is perfectly safe, as long as you take the proper precautions. You can safely carry weights on your wrists, waist, and ankles. Wrist weights are rings that slide over your hand and then snug up on your lower forearm. Start with a half-pound on each wrist. Light weights will not interfere with your smooth rhythm or distort your armswing. Even when you are accustomed to wrist weights, it is important to stop at two pounds.

With a waist carrier designed to position the weights at your sides, over your hips, you can safely carry up to a maximum of about 20 pounds in that position. However, postural distortion and injury can be caused by carrying weights on your abdomen or lower back. Some people like ankle weights. You can safely use very light ones (starting with a half-pound, going up to a maximum of two pounds), as long as you respond appropriately to any unusual pain that develops.

Pace walking with weights in an unsupported pack on your upper back is not recommended. In that position, the weight can constrict both your arm movement and your breathing and distort your posture, leading to injury. You might ask, "But what about hikers, who carry 70 pounds or more on their backs?" The answer is that they are wearing specially designed packs with frames that actually balance most of that weight on their hips.

We do not recommend hand weights. If you squeeze your fingers around the handles, you may cause your blood pressure to increase. Also, if you lose your grip, the weight could fly out of your hand, causing injury to yourself or others.

Effort. People of every age can pace walk. But pace walking is not a magic potion, a single shot that will make you healthy and lean. To bring about its many benefits requires energy, effort, exertion, and commitment.

Even with so natural an exercise as pace walking, you may experience some mild pain, usually of two types. If you are a beginning exerciser, you will encounter some natural stiffness and morning-after pain as you work muscles you may not have used since childhood. If you follow the Take Control plan, which eases you into pace walking very slowly, you should not experience too much of this kind of discomfort.

Once you have established a regular schedule, you may experience some mild pain in your legs, upper arms, and shoulders during your workouts. These pains result from muscle exertion, but have little in common with the more serious pain that accompanies running or from the burn in the thighs that bikers experience pedaling up a steep hill. Experiencing some mild pain while pace walking is perfectly normal.

Other Major Sports

In addition to pace walking, the major sports used for regular exercise are running, cycling, swimming, and aerobic dance and its variants. The minor regular exercise sports are cross-country skiing, rowing, aerobic weight training, and circuit training. Many of these sports and activities can be done in and out of doors. (Both major and minor categories were determined on the basis of numbers of participants and general accessibility.)

Running

Running, once clearly the most popular sport for regular exercise, is familiar to most people. At all but the slowest of speeds it is aerobic. Like pace walking, running requires little monetary investment, is time efficient, and readily accessible. Many people run outdoors, in any kind of weather and during all four seasons. However, you can run indoors at health clubs and gyms that have tracks. You can also run on a motorized treadmill, either at home or at a health club.

If you are curious about the difference between running and jogging, the only important distinction is the one found in the mind of the athlete: if you think of yourself as a runner, then you are a runner, regardless of how fast you move.

Running at a reasonable pace for no more than three to four hours a week while wearing shoes that fit and are in good condition provides you with an exercise program you can pursue without risking serious injury. But people sometimes run for too long at too fast a pace. Or they are careless about their shoes. When they sustain injuries, they blame the sport.

Basic running technique is simple. It is important to keep your body relaxed, your back comfortably but not rigidly straight, shoulders dropped, elbows comfortably bent, fingers lightly closed, with fists not clenched. For the footstrike, land on the heel, not the sole or ball of your foot. Roll forward along the outside edge of the foot, then spring forward off the ball of your foot into the next stride. You should aim for smoothness, rhythm, and balance.

Cycling

Cycling is an exhilarating sport that you can use as part of your regular exercise program. With proper technique, the risk of intrinsic injury is low; but attention to safety is a major consideration for any cyclist because the extrinsic injury risk is the highest of any of the aerobic sports.

As enjoyable as cycling can be, you need to work fairly hard to make sure that the exercise is aerobic. To glide along at 8 to 10 miles per hour is easy, but most people need to ride at a minimum 13 to 15 miles per hour to achieve and maintain an aerobic heart rate.

It is certainly possible to spend a great deal of money on a road bike, but you need not do so in order to enjoy the sport.

Safe outdoor cycling requires safe, accessible roads on which to ride; unfortunately, such roads are not available to everyone. But you can ride indoors, at home or in a health club, on a stationary bicycle, or on a road bike set up on an indoor trainer (a device on which you mount a road bike and ride it against resistance). As with outdoor cycling, you must concentrate to make sure that you are doing the sport intensively enough to gain the desired benefit from it. Whether you ride indoors only when the weather is cold and wet, or you do it as your principal sport, indoor riding has the advantage of being safe, secure, and protected.

Good cycling technique is complex. Learning it requires instruction, time, and practice. Most important is *cadence,* the cyclists' term for pedal revolutions per minute (rpm). The most efficient way to bike is using a high cadence in a low gear. For beginners, this means moving your pedals in the 60–70 rpm range, though the low gear will have you moving along the road at a much lower speed. With experience, you will easily be able to work up to the 80–90 rpm range, which is called *spinning.* Road racers generally try to stay in the 90–105 rpm range. Doing the opposite, using higher gears to get higher road speed with lower pedal speed, results in putting a heavy load on your legs, an invitation to knee problems. Avoid it.

Your upper body should be relaxed. Scrunched-up shoulders will eventually cause pain across your upper back. Your elbows should be comfortably bent. That will help to absorb road shock. Most beginning cyclists ride with their hands on the tops, the crossbar part of the handlebars where the auxiliary brake handles are located on 10-speed bikes. Get rid of the auxiliary brake handles if your bike has them. In sudden stops, auxiliary brake handles may cause confusion that could lead to injury. There are two correct riding positions for your hands on the 10-speed bike: on the hoods that cover the brake handles, and on the drops, the lower curved parts of the handlebars.

As your speed increases on a bike, you spend an increasing amount of energy moving air out of your way. Thus the lower down you get over the handlebars, the more efficiently you will ride, but unless you're going to race, don't be talked into having your seat raised and your handlebars lowered to get your back into an almost horizontal position. If you're cycling only for exercise, and not to see how much distance you can travel, the additional drag created by a more upright position may contribute to the vigor of your workout and will surely add to your enjoyment of the scenery (see the Exercise section in Suggested Readings and General References).

Swimming

Swimming causes none of the pounding, twisting, and jarring associated with running, because the water supports most of your weight, easing the strain on muscles, joints, and heart. Although swimming is mainly an upper-body sport, your lower body also gets a workout, especially if you use breast or side strokes or the trudgen crawl, which combines the crawl stroke with a scissors kick.

For weight loss, swimming has its limitations. Almost all swimming is done in water that has a lower temperature than body temperature, even water in a heated pool. Although the reasons are not completely understood, the adaptation of the body to lower water temperatures apparently inhibits the metabolism of fat.

Nevertheless, swimming is good exercise and can be a good beginner sport for very overweight people. Despite its limitations in a weight-loss program, swimming once or twice a week can be a good part of a cross-training program.

Most swimmers use pools. This limits swimming as a regular exercise because of limited access to a pool and the need to adhere to the pool's schedule. Swimming in a lake or ocean has its own problems: availability, safety (e.g., the possible presence of boats), water conditions, and temperature. But open-water swimming provides a feeling of freedom that is found in few other sports. Assuming you are a reasonably competent swimmer and adhere to proper water-safety rules, open-water swimming is a physically safe sport with a fairly low level of intrinsic injury risk.

Good swimming technique takes time and practice to perfect. Smoothness, rhythm, proper breathing, arm position through the stroke, and leg position are absolutely essential in this sport. Most exercise swimmers use the free-style or

Australian crawl, but you can use the side, breast, or back stroke, as long as you do it aerobically.

If you don't know how to swim but want to learn, find a local YMCA or health club that offers swimming lessons. It's difficult to learn to swim using a book. Some people must overcome fears of drowning, and bad swimming habits are easily developed. Personal instruction can help conquer these problems. However, if you already swim and want to improve your technique, a book can be useful (see Suggested Readings and General References, page 201).

Working out in water at standing depth is enjoyed as a regular exercise by many people. One early proponent, Dr. Jane Katz, calls it the "Water Exercise Technique." Consisting of a series of calisthenic and aerobic dancelike exercises done rhythmically in the water, its advantages are the same as swimming: the water provides support for the body's weight and a gentle resistance to motion. Like swimming, it provides some privacy for the overweight person who is shy about exposing his or her body at the beginning of an exercise program. A number of health clubs and Ys offer regularly scheduled sessions of water exercise, or, you can use one of the available books to set up your own program.

Aerobic Dance

Aerobic dance and its many variations are among the most popular aerobic sports for women, and for an increasing number of men. An activity that can be done in a health club or at home, it has no element of competition. It involves the whole body, and it is aerobic. If done in moderation, particularly using low-impact techniques, it has a relatively low injury risk. Aerobic dance has the least potential for boredom of any of the aerobic sports, especially when done in groups.

An increasingly popular variation of aerobic dance is *stepping,* using a low-level platform on which a wide variety of stepping up and down exercises are performed. The best way to learn aerobic dance or any of its variations is to join a class at a health club or watch and follow a videotape at home. A videotape has the added advantage of instant replay. Books can be helpful too, but you really have to watch someone in action to follow the steps.

Additional Sports

Cross-country skiing, rowing, weight lifting, other muscle exercises against resistance, and circuit training are considered minor sports or activities only because relatively few people use them for regular exercise programs.

Cross-Country Skiing

A truly total body activity, cross-country skiing is probably the best sport for regular exercise. It is smooth and rhythmic, like cycling, and avoids the pounding associated with running. Like running, however, it is almost always aerobic, unless you cross-country ski at a very slow pace. In its outdoor version, it is refreshing and invigorating. Unfortunately, cross-country snow skiing is accessible on a regular basis to very few people.

If you have access to snow and decide to try it, get instructions at the beginning. Entry-level cross-country skiing is not difficult, but it is a good idea to learn the technique from those who are experienced. Although the risk of injury is lower than in downhill skiing, some risk still exists.

More accessible, and engaged in by an increasing number of people, is indoor cross-country skiing using a machine. Several available machines will give you an invigorating workout. An instructor is not needed. The manual that is included with the machine contains all the directions you need to use the machine successfully. And remember, it is virtually impossible to fall off a ski machine.

Rowing

Rowing has much in common with cross-country skiing, in both its disadvantages and advantages. Rowing is aerobic, smooth, rhythmic, and has a fairly low intrinsic injury risk. Rowing a scull on open water requires some skill and practice. In addition, sculls are expensive, and you must face significant problems of access, time, and limitations of the seasons. If you decide to try open-water rowing, be safe and take instruction.

As with cycling and cross-country skiing, you can row indoors for less money, and eliminate the problem of access. Indoor rowing is an excellent sport, and like the cross-country ski machine, the rowing machine will provide a complete workout. There are three kinds of machines: *piston, oarlock* (with friction or piston resistance), and *flywheel*. Stay away from machines that offer "rowing plus"; this term should alert you that compromises in quality may have been made in both the rowing and other exercise parts of the machine.

The most important aspect of rowing technique is to use your whole body. For each stroke, with your back straight, begin by pushing with your legs, then pull through with your shoulders and upper arms. Do not rock back and forth at your waist, since that can cause backstrain.

Weight Training

Weight training can be done aerobically, whether with machines or free weights; it depends upon the routine you use. Body builders and power lifters generally do not work out aerobically. They are interested in lifting large amounts of weight for each rep (repetition) of the exercise in the set (the group of reps taken together). The result is increased muscle strength and bulk. For body builders, the key is high weight, low reps, low sets. However, if you lift low weight for high reps in multiple sets, and do not stop between sets, you can make the workout aerobic. At the same time, you will be increasing muscle flexibility and endurance.

Weight lifting can be done at home or in a gym. For safety reasons, unless you have a partner at home, lifting with free weights (barbells and dumbbells) should be done only in a gym, and only after receiving appropriate instruction. If you are unable to support a weight, you might seriously injure yourself trying to take it down, or worse, dropping it. In contrast, lifting on machines can be safely done on your own. But if you buy a home machine, you should get some instruction in its use before you begin your program. You can find many available books on the many kinds of weight lifting (see Suggested Readings and General References).

Circuit Training

Circuit training is an aerobic sport, perhaps more appropriately termed an *aerobic routine,* found in some health clubs. Because of the high cost and large space needed to set up this kind of training, it is restricted to a gym or club. A circuit of stations is assembled in a row or a circle. At each station you are required to do an exercise. Sometimes the exercises alternate between an aerobic one and some form of weight lifting on a machine. You go through the circuit, doing the exercises in order, on a schedule, which may be monitored for you by a recorded voice broadcast through overhead speakers. You can repeat the circuit as many times as you wish, to give yourself a workout of the length you need for that day.

EQUIPMENT

To enjoy and use a sport for regular exercise, it is not necessary to spend a lot of money. Unless you decide that you simply must have your own swimming pool, there are only two pieces of aerobic sports equipment on which you can spend truly large sums of money: outdoor bicycles and home weight-training devices and equipment.

It is usually not good practice to buy aerobic sports equipment in department stores; you will rarely find well-informed salespeople there. And well-informed sales people are critically important in helping you select the equipment that is right for you. A general sporting goods store, the kind that outfits the local high school football team, may have salespeople who are knowledgeable about running, pace walking, and aerobic dance shoes, but that is not always the case.

Buy your first pair of walking, running, or aerobic dance shoes from a store that specializes in them. Only you can decide what fits comfortably and appeals to you, but the salesperson is usually very familiar with the product and able to give you proper advice on fit and the characteristics of the various shoes that the store sells. Many running-shoe stores are staffed by people who are themselves aerobic athletes, can speak to you from personal experience, and can pass on comments of other users of a particular shoe.

Shoes

For most sports, the single most important item of equipment is shoes. Some shoe advertisements would have you believe that the right shoe will convert an ordinary athlete into a superstar, an absurd contention. But the action of virtually all the sports discussed in this book, except swimming, begins with the feet. The right shoe making contact between you and the pavement, floor, or pedal can make a world of difference for avoiding injury and being comfortable.

Shoes appropriate for any sport share several characteristics. First, the shoe must fit well; that is, it should touch your foot in as many places as possible except over the toes. Conversely, the toe box itself should be roomy—to allow your foot to roll naturally. In other words, a good sport shoe fits like a glove with no fingers. Second, the shoe must be comfortable. Although your foot should fit snugly in the shoe, it should not be pinched, squeezed, or squashed at any point. The shoe should not cause any pain or discomfort when you are standing or moving. Third, people who overpronate (a common problem in which people roll their ankles too far inward with each step) have special problems and should buy shoes designed to resist overpronation. Uncorrected, the condition can easily lead to injury higher up the leg. Less frequent a problem is supination—the ankle rolls outward with each step. A few shoes are designed to control this condition also.

Finally, the shoe should be specifically designed for the sport in which you are engaging. Aerobic dance shoes give you the cushioning flexibility and ease of lateral motion you need for aerobic dancing. Walking shoes provide cushioning, support, and forward, not lateral, flexibility. But walking shoes will not work well for aerobic dance.

Monitoring wear in shoes is very important to prevent injury. Deciding when your shoes should be replaced can be tricky, but it is better to discard a pair of shoes too soon than too late. How do you know when the time has come to replace shoes? Most quality running, walking, and aerobic dance shoes have a midsole, the material sandwiched between the outside tread and the bottom of the foot compartment. Midsole material is compressible. The midsoles in most running shoes will develop horizontal lines as they are used, and as the cushioning material becomes permanently compressed. Learn the feel of the shoe when it is new and check those lines periodically. Too many lines means the midsole has become overcompressed (how many is too many is something you will have to learn from experience). When the midsole becomes overcompressed the shoe will no longer provide adequate cushioning, which can lead to injury.

As a rule, if you are running two to three hours a week in quality shoes, you should examine your midsoles after three months of wear. If there are many lines, or if the shoe appears to be developing a tilt to one side when looked at from the back, it's time to visit the running-shoe store to have a specialist check your shoes.

Because specialists are best equipped to help you obtain the right fit and function, it is wise to buy your first pair of walking/running/aerobic-exercise shoes from a specialized athletic footwear store, rather than from a department store, mail-order house, or a sneaker shop.

Walking shoes. The forefoot of the walking shoe, the part that runs from the toe to the ball of your foot, should be flexible. A flexible forefoot will allow a full follow-through with each step as you walk. Remember that it's the follow-through that provides the lift that's such a nice part of exercise walking. Once you've increased your speed, you may find running shoes more comfortable than walking shoes, because the former generally tend to have a more flexible forefoot. There should be adequate cushioning under the heel, but the walking shoe heelstrike is not nearly as hard as in running, so you won't need the cushioning of a top-of-the-line running shoe.

Your foot should feel secure within the shoe. To help achieve this, there should be a firm *heel counter,* the hard piece of material in the back of the shoe that fits around your heel. Movement of your foot inside the shoe can produce both blisters and musculoskeletal injury, so the heel counter, combined with a good fit, must keep your foot from slipping around inside the shoe. The shoe's outersole should be designed to flex forward easily as your foot rolls over it, while limiting lateral motion.

Most major running-shoe manufacturers offer one or more models of exercise walking shoe, a sign that pace walking is now accepted as a serious aerobic sport.

Running shoes. Running shoes are generally designed to provide heel cushioning, heel support, and a modest degree of forefoot flexibility. The heavier runner needs more cushioning and support. For the overpronator, more resistive material is built into the shoe along its inside edge. For supinators, it's on the outside edge. Otherwise, the general comments on all athletic shoes also apply to running shoes.

Aerobic dance/exercise shoes. Aerobic dance/exercise shoes need to have a substantial amount of cushioning under the ball of the foot, which is where you land in most of the routines. Some experts believe ankle support is also a necessary feature of aerobic dance shoes, to prevent the foot from rolling over. The tread of the outer sole should be designed to allow for lateral motion. Otherwise, the general comments on shoes apply.

There are some general aerobic fitness or cross-training shoes on the market, advertised as being good for use in all of the generally aerobic sports. Although they may be suitable for all those sports, they do not provide the optimum performance for any one activity. With the widely varying requirements among the different aerobic sports, it would be very difficult to design a shoe that is suitable for all of them.

Bicycling shoes. Although the shoe is not the most important piece of equipment in cycling, it is important. If you cycle seriously, you will use toe clips on the pedals. Toe clips keep your foot firmly attached to the pedal on the upstroke. As you learn to ride, you will find that the upstroke is as useful in making your bike go forward as the downstroke. Thus bike shoes are designed to fit into toe clips, and are held in place by a small cleat attached to the sole of the foot. In the late 1980s, quick-release clipless pedal systems were developed. These make riding with your shoes cleated to the pedals much easier and safer.

In contrast to walking/running/aerobic-exercise shoes, bike shoes all have rigid soles. The soles of touring shoes run from the heel to the ball of the foot, in racing shoes from heel to toe. The rigid sole keeps your foot flat during the downstroke on the pedal. If your heel bends on the downstroke you lose power. The design of touring shoes makes it possible for you to walk in them.

Walking in a racing shoe is very limited, not only because of the full-length stiff sole, but also because the protruding cleat tilts you back on your heels.

Although the touring shoe doesn't attach your foot as firmly to the pedal as does the racing shoe, even when the former is used with a toe clip, you may find it an acceptable compromise for your first cycling shoe.

A recent product in the cycling-shoe market is the mountain bike shoe, really a rugged touring shoe with a recessed cleat for use with a quick-release locking pedal. This combines most of the advantages of the racing shoe (although it is not as light and cool) with a somewhat flexible forefoot and the capability of walking.

You should not use walking or running shoes for cycling, unless you are using pedals without toe clips. Such shoes tend to have wide soles that can be difficult to put into toe clips and even more difficult to take out, especially in an emergency. Furthermore, their flexible soles cause power loss, as noted above. Whatever shoes you buy for cycling, you should purchase them in a bike shop, from a knowledgeable salesperson.

Bicycles

The most important design requirements for a bike are that it have a sturdy yet lightweight frame (steel or aluminum alloy rather than straight steel, even if it is described as high-tensile steel) and aluminum alloy wheels. These days, most of the better bikes come with indexed, click-stop, shift mechanisms that make shifting gears much easier and more precise than the old friction shift system you may remember from the 10-speed you rode as a child.

The all-steel frames on the inexpensive bikes are heavy, uncomfortable, and unresponsive. The wheels and tires are heavy and offer much rolling resistance. The shift mechanisms are heavy, clunky, and difficult to work properly, especially on hills. You will get a very good workout in terms of the effort that you have to invest to make the bike go, but you won't have as much fun, and probably will soon stop riding.

If you can afford to buy a quality bike, the difference in the superiority of the frame and components is usually worth it. Delay buying one of the more expensive bikes with super-light steel alloy, aluminum, or carbon-fiber frames until you know that you really like cycling.

Always wear a helmet when riding. If you fall off your bike and hit your head on the ground or pavement, you'll know the investment was well worth it. Make sure the helmet you select is either ANSI or Snell certified. These certifications indicate that the helmet has been proven to offer maximum level of protection in the event of a fall. Make sure, too, that you can adjust the straps so that the helmet can't be pushed off your head. If you find you can't adjust the helmet, exchange it for another model.

Many bikes come with attachments for a water-bottle carrier. If you plan to ride for any distance (more than 30 minutes), carry a water bottle.

Indoor exercise bike. When purchasing an indoor exercise bike look for the following: a well-built, rigid frame; a heavy, weighted flywheel that is truly round, with the ability to coast like a road bike so that you get a smooth ride; well-placed, easy-to-work controls; a well-padded seat that is easy to adjust; readable instruments; and toe straps so that you can power the upstroke as well as the downstroke.

Before investing in an indoor bicycle, you should be sure that you will use the device regularly and over a long period of time. As noted previously, you can also mount a road bike on an indoor trainer. If you own a road bike and want to ride indoors in the winter, a trainer is obviously the cheapest solution. However, for some people a road bike on a trainer may not provide as comfortable a ride as an indoor exercise bike. And the exposed chain and wheel spokes pose a hazard to children's fingers.

Stopwatch. You will need a stopwatch to time your workouts, check your heart rate, and count your cadence on the bike if it is not equipped with a computer. A digital watch with the right features can be used for this purpose.

Weight-Training Machines

Many weight-lifting machines are available for home use. They are designed to provide a variety of exercises through changes in cable-and-pulley arrangements and attachments.

Look for the following characteristics in a quality multistation machine that you can use safely at home: welded, rather than bolted, main joints (bolted main joints eventually work loose); if the machine uses cables and pulleys, both should be made entirely of steel (aluminum cable and plastic pulleys wear easily); if it uses rubber bands, or springs, or hydraulic mechanisms, it is difficult to judge quality, but they should at least appear to be well made; a well-padded bench; enough different stations to give you a thorough workout with variety. Even with a weight-lifting machine, you can injure yourself by lifting too much weight or lifting the wrong way. But since the resistance in a machine is provided either by weights sliding on a track or by bands or pistons, it is highly unlikely that you will incur the type of crushing injury that can happen occasionally with free weights.

As with any expensive piece of equipment, you should be convinced that you are going to use a weight-training machine over the long term before you purchase it. First join a reputable health club that has a weight-training program and qualified instructors, for a three-month trial membership. Decide if you like weight training. If you do, you may decide to stick with the club. Or you can purchase a quality machine with confidence that you will enjoy weight training.

Choosing a Health Club

In one sense a health club is a collection of equipment you rent for a period of time. There are, however, guidelines to help you select one. The club should be reasonably close to home, easy to reach, and, if you will be driving to it, have plenty of adjacent, safe parking space. The hours should be convenient. The locker rooms and the workout areas should be clean and well lighted.

The club should have the facilities and activities in which you are interested. Most will have free weights, at least one type of weight-machine circuit, exercise bicycles, and various kinds of aerobics classes. Many now have cross-country ski machines, stair climbers, rowing machines, treadmills, and circuit training. There should be enough equipment and classes to accommodate members without a long wait during peak periods. The more elaborate clubs will have an indoor track and may have a lap swimming pool.

There should also be adequate staff. By the nature of their jobs the staff will be eager to sell you a membership, but they should also be knowledgeable, experienced, and interested in helping you. Inquire about safety and the availability of staff trained in cardiopulmonary resuscitation (CPR). Find out how many of the staff are certified in exercise supervision by one of several certifying organizations, such as the American College of Sports Medicine, the Aerobics and Fitness Association of America, the International Dance-Exercise Association, or the Institute for Aerobics Research. If individual trainers are available, almost always at extra cost, ask about their qualifications.

Many types of memberships are available. Be sure to ask what specials are being offered. Check your local newspapers and weekly giveaways for special-price coupons. Some clubs offer very attractive rates if you make use of them only during off-peak hours. While most clubs like to sign you up for a long-term contract, an increasing number offer pay-by-the month or short-term trial memberships. In general, the longer the term you choose, the less expensive it will be on a weekly basis. Don't sign a contract on your first visit to the first club you visit. Check out several, and try to get the best deal.

Clothing

Regular exercise and aerobic sports clothing is something that you can spend a lot of money on, but you don't have to. You can probably assemble a basic wardrobe for your sport of choice out of your closet and dresser. Clothing should be loose-fitting and comfortable. It is generally recommended that you wear socks to help avoid blisters. For women a jogging bra is recommended. Men should wear support briefs or an athletic supporter under their shorts. An increasing number of men and women are wearing bike shorts (without the seat padding if you are not planning to bike) for a wide variety of indoor and outdoor sports.

For cold-weather outdoor exercise, use several layers of light-to-moderate-weight garments rather than one heavyweight set. You want clothing that breathes, that allows the moisture to wick through the fabric and evaporate. Heavy cotton sweats retain the moisture. As moisture condenses and drips onto your skin, it makes you feel colder, not warmer.

On a chilly day, you should wear enough clothing to feel cool when starting out. If you feel warm at the beginning of a workout on a cold day, you are sure to feel hot and uncomfortable well before the end of it. Polypropylene, capilene, and other materials designed to wick moisture off your skin are best to wear next to your skin. The most useful outer layer is made of breathable fabrics. These fabrics have billions of tiny pores in them that let moisture escape yet also keep cold air out. A polypropylene layer next to the skin, a breathable fabric outer garment, a warm hat, and gloves can make pace walking in winter very enjoyable.

NOTE TO THE READER

In the final analysis, the Take Control of Your Weight philosophy is about *choice*. If you are overweight, you can certainly choose to stay that way. But you have the power to change your body weight and shape if you Take Control. If you are making a choice that will work for you for the rest of your life, your choice needs to be an informed one. I hope this book has been useful in providing you with reliable information and advice in which you can have confidence.

If you do identify your pathway to overweight and, using the information in this book, have chosen the pathway back to losing those unwanted pounds and keeping them off, and have found that this method works for you, I would like to hear from you. Please send a letter describing your weight-loss experiences to:

Steven Jonas, M.D., M.P.H.
c/o Consumer Reports Books
101 Truman Avenue
Yonkers, NY 10703-1057

Of course, if the book has *not* been helpful to you, or if you have any suggestions for improving my weight-loss program, please let me know. Your firsthand experiences may be of help to the readers of future editions of this book. Unfortunately, I will not be able to acknowledge each letter individually, but if you respond to this request, you have my heartfelt thanks in advance.

APPENDIX A

Risks and Benefits of
Obesity and Weight Loss

OBESITY* carries with it a number of health risks. Risks are not certainties. It is not a certainty that being obese will cause you to experience any of the negative conditions associated with excessive weight. The only certainty is that obesity significantly increases your *chances* of incurring certain illnesses or conditions, such as diabetes or hypertension. The Take Control of Your Weight Program presupposes that it is your individual choice whether to accept the risks or to do something about them.

Just how overweight a person must be before any significant health risks occur is debatable. Overweight that is less than 20 percent above the upper end of the normal range for your age (see Table I.1 on page 9) does not seem to carry perceptible health risks. There are health risks associated with mild (20 to 40 percent above) and moderate (41 to 100 percent above) overweight, which are not always proportional to the degree of overweight. Certainly severe or morbid obesity (more than double the upper end of the normal range) always carries a measurable increase in health risk, and a decrease in longevity.

Physical Health Risks of Obesity

In many cases, obesity increases the risk of dying before reaching normal life expectancy. For example, adult-onset diabetes is three times more common in obese people than in those whose weight is within the normal range. Diabetes can cause damage to the kidneys, eyes, nerves, and blood vessels, the last con-

---

Obesity is the word generally used in risk-factor literature, so we are using obesity instead of overweight in this particular section. Readers should also know that obesity in the sense it is used here means obesity at the level that increases health risks.

dition secondarily increasing the risk of heart attack and stroke. Obesity can lead to this kind of diabetes by making the body's tissues resistant to the sugar-processing action of insulin.

For reasons that are not entirely clear, obesity increases the risk of hypertension. It also causes an increase in the serum level of cholesterol, a fatty substance that normally circulates in the blood. (Blood serum, by the way, is the yellowish fluid that's left over when the blood clots.) An elevated serum cholesterol level can lead to narrowing of the blood vessels because of the extra fatty substances being deposited in their walls. That condition, called *atherosclerosis,* can lead to significant heart and brain damage, among other things.

Obesity also causes an increase in the level of triglycerides, another fatty substance that normally circulates in the blood. This can lead to the accumulation of extra fat in the blood, which usually results in extra fat in the liver. Extra fat can interfere with liver function, which is to manufacture the majority of all internal chemicals we need in order to survive. Obesity also increases the risk of gallstones, which are formed from some of the body's food-processing chemicals and waste materials. Gallstones accumulate in the gallbladder, a small storage sac attached to the liver, and cause inflammation of the gallbladder or obstruction to the flow of bile.

Diabetes, hypertension, and elevated serum cholesterol all increase the risk of a heart attack. Also, a large amount of extra weight can increase the physical burden on the heart, causing it to pump extra blood, which may lead to enlargement of the heart and heart failure. The risk of stroke is increased by both atherosclerosis and hypertension, both complications of obesity. Certain kinds of cancers have been linked to obesity—cancers of the colon, rectum, prostate, and one type of cancer of the uterus—though the causal linkage to these diseases has not yet been fully established. Obesity also increases the risk of developing several of the possible complications of pregnancy.

Two kinds of arthritis are more prevalent among obese people than among people of normal weight. One is gout, a condition caused by an elevation in the blood serum level of uric acid, a body waste chemical. Osteoarthritis, resulting from wear and tear within the joints, is the most common type of arthritis. Excess weight can increase the risk of developing osteoarthritis in the hips, knees, and ankles, as well as in the lower back because of the strain of carrying extra poundage. Finally, obesity harms indirectly by fostering a more sedentary life-style.

In addition to the multiple physical risks associated with obesity, the condition also increases the risk of social and psychological problems.

Benefits of Overweight

The benefits of overweight are generally evolutionary and are related to the ability of humans to store fat. In times of famine, overweight people are more likely to survive than their thinner neighbors. After all, body fat is nothing more than stored energy.

Excess body fat also helps maintain body temperature if you are submerged in cold water for a long period of time. But this would prove useful only if you are a long-distance cold-water swimmer, or if you are shipwrecked—both unlikely situations. Body fat may also protect against osteoporosis, a thinning of the bones, by converting certain weak hormones into estrogen.

Benefits of Losing Weight

The benefits of losing weight are obvious, but are worth restating.

- You feel good physically and feel better about yourself.
- Your appearance is enhanced and clothes fit and look better.
- You feel capable of engaging in regular physical exercise, which is essential if you want to keep the weight off permanently.
- You have reduced your risk of contracting a variety of diseases and negative health conditions associated with overweight.
- You have confidence in your ability to control your body and your life.

These major advantages of losing weight obviously affect your whole life, especially your attitude toward yourself. Are there any disadvantages or risks to losing weight? Surprisingly, yes.

Risks of Losing Weight

The risks of weight loss are psychological: fear of failure and fear of success.

Fear of Failure

If you are trying to lose weight, fear of failure is a major inhibitor. As a chronic dieter, for example, you may have dieted successfully in the past only to regain all the pounds later on. Or you may have had several previous failures, and you don't want to go through that depressing experience again.

Furthermore, you may have the justifiable fear that you will suffer the yo-yo dieting cycle, alternately blowing up and slimming down. Not only is that cycle frustrating and painful, but the physical process itself can be damaging to your health.

Dieting programs. It is difficult to lose weight, and apparently organized dieting programs don't help all that much. To be fair, the low success rate of many weight-loss programs may be related more to the characteristics of the people who join them than to either the metabolic realities of life or the specific food and exercising components of the program. The people who try these structured programs probably have already attempted and failed to lose weight on their own. They may be programmed for failure in one way or another; if the program doesn't deal with these hidden problems, the likelihood is that the person will fail again.

As researchers have discovered about smokers, people who try to lose weight on their own are usually more successful. This evidence suggests that if you have tried in the past to lose weight and have failed, you may succeed if you have the inner motivation to make gradual life-style changes by yourself.

Fear of failure is a very real barrier to losing weight. You will need to confront this fear, deal with it, and convince yourself that the potential benefits of success are worth taking that risk.

Fear of Success

This type of reverse fear may affect some obese people. In general, the fear of losing weight concerns one's emotional and sexual relationships. A few examples will make this clear:

Fred is 38 years old, 5 feet 10 inches tall, and weighs 285 pounds. He has been married and divorced twice. A gourmet chef who understands and loves food, he lost his first wife because she could not adjust to his working at night. His second wife had left him after he had gained a great deal of weight. She said she didn't want to be married to a fat man.

Fred knows he should lose weight, knows what to do, and is confident he could do it. But, deep down, he doesn't really want to. He realizes that his present obesity acts as a protection against his getting involved again with a woman. For Fred, staying fat is safer than trying once more to find the "right" person, and having to work hard at maintaining a loving relationship. So he remains heavy, unhappy but managing to avoid stress and psychological upset.

Charlotte is another example. At age 43, the mother of three teenage children, she was recently divorced. Charlotte is 5 feet 4 inches tall, and now weighs 193 pounds. She had begun putting on weight after the birth of her second child. She had lost the pounds on several occasions in the past, but that did not improve her marriage.

Nevertheless, Charlotte would like to be in a truly loving relationship, but now she is afraid to try. Staying overweight seems far more comfortable. She can concentrate on being a busy, loving mother, avoiding the possibility of stressful sexual and emotional entanglements.

Obviously, no one can persuade Fred or Charlotte to lose weight. Both must confront their fears and decide freely if obesity is the right solution for them. Perhaps it is—unless and until something happens that persuades them otherwise and they develop the inner motivation to change.

APPENDIX B

Being Overweight:

The Psychosocial Factors

CONTEMPORARY American society has a powerful influence on our physical self-perception and personal priorities. A leading authority on weight loss, Dr. Kelly Brownell, puts it very well:

> Modern society breeds a search for the perfect body. Today's aesthetic ideal is extremely thin, and now, superimposed on this, is a need to be physically fit. People seek the ideal, not only because of expected health benefits, but because of what the ideal symbolizes in our culture (self-control, success, acceptance). Two assumptions are widespread with regard to body weight and shape. One is that the body is infinitely malleable, and that with the right combination of diet and exercise, every person can reach the ideal. The second is that vast rewards await the person who attains the ideal. Research has shown that biological variables, particularly genetics, are influential in the regulation of body weight and shape. Hence, there are limits to how much a person can change.*

Dr. Brownell points out that in the search for the perfect body Americans spend about $30 billion a year on diets and dieting, exercise, and plastic surgery. Most people engaged in this search tend to operate on two widely held assumptions. One is that anybody can approach the established ideal, if only you eat right and exercise, if you work hard enough at it, if you spend enough time, money, and energy doing it. The other is that thinness has great rewards,

*K. D. Brownell, "Dieting and the Search for the Perfect Body," *Behavior Therapy* 22 (1991):1–12.

that if you become slimmer, fitter, and thus more attractive, your life will improve dramatically.

What is the "ideal" body? For most of us, does it bear any resemblance to reality? Dr. Brownell relates a story from *Self* magazine: One of the editors stood 5 foot 7 inches tall and weighed 124 pounds. By most standards she would be considered rather slender. Yet she *felt* herself to be somewhat heavy. So she decided to find out what she would have to do to measure up to that American ideal of womanhood, Barbie of Barbie-doll fame. Applying the doll's relative measurements to herself, she discovered that to achieve the ideal she would have to expand 12 inches in the bust (in the right proportion of course), shrink 10 inches in the waist, and grow to a height of 7 feet 2 inches. If such desires to fit the ideal did not produce so many sad results for so many people, these expectations would be comic indeed.

As Dr. Brownell points out, being thin does not necessarily carry with it great rewards. It might make you more physically attractive to some. But it won't make you smarter or give you a sense of humor or convert you into an interesting conversationalist or make you more adept at sex. Because of our society's emphasis on good looks, a slim body may get you to the starting line more easily in both personal and work relationships. But if you don't have the other qualities necessary for lasting relationships, it will not solve your problem. Conversely, being overweight does not make a smart, funny, interesting, sexy person suddenly become dumb, humorless, dull, and sexless.

The Limits of Body Change

The reason that people don't like what they see in the mirror really has little to do with their physical makeup. Instead, it reflects how they are used to seeing themselves. And because self-esteem is the product of total life experience from childhood on, it is difficult to change low self-esteem to high with surgery, body building, or body reshaping.

In dealing with body image and self-image, it is critically important to remember that your body is *not* infinitely malleable. It is true that virtually anyone can become more physically attractive, to themselves and/or others, by losing some weight or redistributing it, or by adding muscle while shedding fat. And anyone can be changed under the plastic surgeon's knife. But all of us start out with certain genetically programmed body characteristics, such as bone structure and hair distribution. The nature of those characteristics limits how far each individual can go in changing his or her appearance.

Take the singer-actress Cher. She lost weight, built up muscle through exercise, and has had some plastic surgery. But a major reason that Cher is as attractive as many consider her to be is that right from the start she had a certain body shape, facial structure, and proportion of torso and extremities.

Consider the body builder/actor Arnold Schwarzenegger. He spent countless hours building up his muscle mass, and then countless more shaping it and rebalancing it. There are many people who could have spent the same number of hours and not built up such muscle mass, or any at all, because their muscles are simply not genetically capable of "bulking" up.

The societal emphasis on thinness, plus other psychological factors, can lead to mental distortions about body image. Thus a 45-year-old man can be 5 feet 10 inches tall, weigh 170 pounds, and have a 34-inch waist, yet look at himself in the mirror and see flab and fat. Why? Because he doesn't have a very low body-fat proportion (so that muscle definition can be seen through the skin) nor does he have bulging biceps and shoulders that merge imperceptibly into a neck that is as big around as his skull.

Is he truly fat and flabby? By the standards of most people, no. But he may be absolutely convinced that he is flabby, no matter what positive features of his body are pointed out to him. He has a body-image distortion. That is, what he sees when he looks in the mirror does not correspond to reality. Many of us have this problem to some extent, but for most of us the distortion is limited and not harmful. It may even help motivate us to change to a healthier diet, engage in regular exercise, and build up our muscle mass.

But sometimes body-image distortion can get us into trouble. People can become clinically depressed about their bodies, which may lead to physical and mental immobilization. Body-image distortion can also cause an obsession with the body, so that you think about it much of the time and become consumed with correcting its real or imagined flaws. Finally, body-image distortion can lead to serious (even occasionally fatal) eating disorders, such as bulimia and anorexia.

Bulimia and anorexia. In bulimia, people eat a normal or near-normal amount of food, although they spend a great amount of time weighing and measuring portions. What marks them as bulimics is that they will periodically go on eating binges that are followed by vomiting or "purging," using laxatives. Anorexics are also convinced they are fat, and will consume little or nothing at all until they waste away. Many anorexics are also bulimic.

Anorexia and bulimia are not necessarily disorders of eating, per se. They are disorders of self-perception and a failure of self-love. Because they are disorders of perception, persons with these afflictions are never thin enough, no matter how much weight they lose.

If you suspect that you (or a family member or friend) have an eating disorder, don't attempt to try the Take Control of Your Weight Program. Instead, seek the counsel of a registered dietitian/nutritionist or consult your physician immediately.

Fear of Fat

Not only is society's overemphasis on thinness counterproductive, but it has also fomented an element of social prejudice against obese people. This bias manifests itself in a number of ways. As Dr. Lynn Bennion and colleagues point out in *Straight Talk About Weight Control*: "Our society almost always assumes the worst about people who are fat. 'Fatty, fatty, two-by-four,' and 'I don't want her, you can have her, she's too fat for me,' are cruel but common expressions of the prejudice against fat people that pervades our culture."

Some use the word *lipophobia* (fear of fat) to describe the variety of behaviors directed toward obese people, including discrimination in college and university acceptance rates, job discrimination, decreased marriage rates, decreased upward social mobility, even limited selections in clothing and fashion (although this is beginning to change).

Sadly, most of this prejudice is directed at women, which is ironic since the negative health consequences of overweight may be more serious for men. A growing body of scientific evidence points to the fact that excess poundage located around the waist and belly is considerably more harmful than fat around the hips and thighs, a condition more common in women.

Behind the current social stress on the vital importance of thinness for women is the popular notion among lay people that ultimately all overweight is the result of overeating. Unfortunately, many health professionals also still consider overweight to be the result of pure self-indulgence and lack of control.

We now know that many overweight people are *not* overeaters (see chapter 1). Indeed, it is all too possible that millions of the overweight can honestly say "I don't eat, but I can't lose weight." This is because much overweight is produced by the process of dieting itself; excess weight is difficult to modify for genetic reasons or is perhaps caused by irreversible proliferation of the number of fat cells.

In the case of diet-induced overweight, the person tries hard to lose weight, goes too far too fast, and stimulates the starvation response. In such cases, obesity can truly be considered a socially induced condition. (Perhaps we should recognize the concept of a *dieting disorder*.)

Psychological Factors

In the 1950s, the medical community generally believed that obesity was caused by what your mother did to you when you were young, or what was done to your mother when *she* was young, or that it was the manifestation of some severe neurotic problem. More recent psychologists' formulations suggest that, in some cases, being overweight results from a fear of sex, or of relationships, or even of having to make oneself presentable each day. These psychological characterizations of obesity are unproven. Certainly they could apply to some obese people and to many people who are not overweight.

But we do know that the psychological pain resulting from obesity can be intense. As Lynn Bennion, Edwin Bierman, and James Ferguson point out:

> The psychological consequences of obesity range from a mild sense of inferiority to severe incapacitation. . . . For many obese persons contempt for their own bodies, and feelings of guilt, embarrassment, helplessness, and failure brought on by their obesity are more painful than their physical suffering.
>
> As medical research makes it plain that obesity is not someone's "fault," some of the guilt associated with obesity may lessen. On the other hand, until effective long-term treatment becomes available, feelings of helplessness and of the unfairness of fate and society will continue to plague many who suffer from being obese.*

Reactions. It is only natural that excessive societal pressure for thinness has produced a backlash among those who are overweight. This reaction has resulted in a number of claims on the part of some vocal obese people, including:

- The overweight population should give up trying to lose weight and society should stop trying to force them to do so.
- Instead of trying to lose pounds, overweight people should work on self-acceptance and improvement of their self-esteem, learning to accept the bodies they have been given.
- If overweight people are interested in improving their appearance, they should focus on more flattering clothing, makeup, and the like, not on weight or body shape.

*Lynn J. Bennion, Edwin L. Bierman, James M. Ferguson, and the Editors of Consumer Reports Books, *Straight Talk About Weight Control* (Yonkers: Consumer Reports Books, 1991).

Some obese people also claim that the social pressure for thinness is an artificial construct that varies with the times, and has more to do with a male-dominated society's view of women than it does with any real concern about health. They say that genetic or biological reasons make significant weight loss impossible for most people.

A third claim is that diets don't work and, in fact, dieting may instead exacerbate overweight. A fourth opinion is that obesity is not really harmful to health, or is at least not as harmful as many have claimed it is. And further, dieting itself, especially continued up-and-down weight cycling (yo-yo dieting), is more harmful to both physical and mental health than is the original excess weight. Finally, some obese people even express the opinion that weight-loss programs and other treatments/interventions offered to the overweight are nothing more than an exercise in victimization, based on the greed of promoters who know that the possibility for long-term success is very slight.

Taking a Position

Obviously, people should not be discriminated against or ridiculed for being overweight, or censured for their supposed lack of discipline. On the contrary, it seems reasonable to accept obesity as a life-style choice, if only because losing weight is difficult, if not impossible, for many people.

Obesity is a legitimate choice, in the civil liberties sense, so long as that choice is freely made after full consideration of the risks and benefits of obesity and the risks and benefits of the weight-loss process. Losing weight is difficult. At the same time, even after admitting that the prevailing social attitude toward overweight is ignorant and destructive, certain statements of questionable validity regarding obesity have been made by the proponents of an overweight life-style.

Let's look at the facts. Conceding that most calorie-restriction diets don't work, that dieting itself can be a significant cause of overweight, and that yo-yo dieting is a health-risk does not lead inevitably to the conclusion that there are *no* approaches to successful weight loss for many overweight people.

Furthermore, it is true that many overweight people are not overeaters, but some, especially overweight males, *are* overconsumers of calories (an example is the habitual beer drinker). For them, a properly designed and implemented calorie-restrictive eating program has a good chance of leading to significant weight loss.

Although some organized weight-loss programs, such as some of the very-low-calorie diets (VLCDs), can truly be considered as nothing more than exercises in victimization based on greed, not all weight-loss programs should be lumped into that category. Nor should one have to accept false statements such as "It is not true that if you move around, you won't be fat, because exercise has little real effect on your weight." The scientific evidence is very sound that regular exercise is a key element in weight loss, especially if you have diet-induced low-calorie overweight.

Let's look at the present state of scientific thinking on overweight. As a risk factor, overweight below the 20 percent line is usually not considered harmful to physical health in any measurable way. There is also disagreement over how much and what kinds of health risks are associated with mild or moderate obesity. However, morbid obesity is generally thought to carry very measurable health risks. Distortions of the scientific evidence cannot help the "fat is okay" movement, just as the supermarket tabloid's "lose 20 pounds in 10 days" diet does not promote health and successful weight loss.

APPENDIX C

Benefits of Racing

REGULAR EXERCISE is part of the program many people follow in order to lose weight. Usually they find exercise enjoyable but some never consider it more than an adjunct to weight loss and maintenance. Many other people, however, find that regular exercise becomes the focal point of their daily activities, and they become interested in distance sport racing.

There are many reasons to try racing after you've established a reasonable aerobic base. Racing is just plain fun, so long as the race you choose is of reasonable length and you don't overdo it. Moreover, races are colorful affairs that are usually held in pleasant weather; the atmosphere is generally happy and expectant. Racers are fun to meet and talk with, and most are not overly competitive. Many of them are there just to run the race, not to win. Of course, if you have the ability to win, fine, but don't worry if you don't. Most road racers do not race against other entrants; they race *with* them. There are no opponents, simply the boundaries of your own body and mind.

When you finish your first race, whatever your distance and time, you'll feel a special sense of accomplishment. If you decide to tackle longer distances, you'll experience those feelings again as you pass each milestone. Racing can expand your mental limits, and give you an understanding of yourself that you never had before.

Racing can also serve as a focus and catalyst for your exercise training. Each year you can plan a racing schedule for the months ahead and set up your training schedule around it. This approach is useful regardless of the length of the races you run or walk.

For example, you decide to pace walk a 5-kilometer (3.1 miles) or a 10-kilometer (6.2 miles) running road race. (Yes, it's perfectly legitimate for pace walkers to enter running races. The organizers will be happy to collect your entry fee, and you may finish ahead of the slower runners.) Give yourself plenty of time to train, choose a date, and find a nearby race. Use the Maintenance Plus or Double Plus Take Control Exercise Plan (see chapter 8) to set up a suitable training schedule for yourself.

If you enjoy the first race, try another one soon after. Space out your races and set up your training program around them. Before you realize it, training will have become a means to an end.

Of course, racing is not for everyone. For example, some people find that in a race their competitive instincts get the better of them. When they don't win, they feel depressed and stressed out, and soon they are grimly training with only the race in mind. If this pattern continues, they don't enjoy the racing or the training, thus canceling out the benefits of both activities.

Types of Races

Many kinds of races are open to the regular exerciser. Running and walking are the most popular forms of sport racing. Road-race distances range from 1 mile to 100 miles, although the most common are 5 miles, 10 miles, 12.4 miles, half-marathon (13.1 miles), and marathon (26.2 miles).

Race walkers can also find contests organized just for them. These racers are judged for adherence to race walking rules, so you have to be familiar with race walking techniques to perform properly in these races. You don't have to worry about speed, though. While a top race walker can do a mile in 7 minutes, many competitors are in the 12 to 14 minutes-per-mile range.

You can locate running and walking races through local shoe and sporting goods stores, private clubs, and the national and local running and walking magazines and newsletters that are distributed through these stores and at your local newsstand. Check your community recreation center for the dates of local races.

There are other types of competitions, too. Many local bicycle clubs run entry-level bike races of various distances. Look for notices in your neighborhood bicycle pro shop. Races for master swimmers (that is, swimmers over age 25) are held in many areas of the country. Look for them at your local Y, or scan the bulletin boards at a college or university pool that is open to the community. Multiple competitions, such as triathlons and duathlons, are posted at local bike and sports stores, or check the listings in the national monthlies *Triathlon Today!* and *Triathlete.* Regional supplements listing nearly every local race in the nation can be found in *Triathlon Today!*

Races are organized by clubs, businesses, churches and synagogues, hospitals, schools, universities, volunteer fire departments, charities, health agencies, and private entrepreneurs. If you are uncertain about competing, try volunteering your services to help organize a race. You can handle registration, be a course marshal, or operate the first-aid and water stations. You'll get a feel for the sport and have a good view of things from the inside track.

Setting Up a Pace-Walking Club and Contest

YOU CAN MAKE regular exercise fun by doing it with others, at least for some of your usual workouts. One easy way to find partners is by joining an exercise club. You can locate such clubs through your chamber of commerce or local village, town, and county recreation departments.

If this type of club isn't available in your community, consider forming one. It's not difficult, but does take an investment of time and a modest degree of commitment both to your own exercise program and one that includes organized activities for others.

The following organizational scheme uses pace walking as the prototype sport, but the advice would work for setting up any type of exercise group.

Establish Your Goals

When organizing an exercise club, you must first have a clear grasp of the club's purposes. Goals can include:

- Scheduling regular aerobic exercise workouts for yourself and others
- Finding other pace walkers who have similar goals and knowledge of the sport
- Providing social opportunities for members who have a common interest in exercise and health
- Offering a means of exchange of information on varied aspects of health and fitness
- Taking trips designed to include regular pace walking and other exercise
- Organizing pace walking races and contests
- Entering your group in particular races, whether pace walking or running competitions

A pace-walking club can provide a central focus to members who want to lose weight; a club also offers mutual support and advice. Whatever your goals, if they are clearly established from the outset, you have a good chance of setting up a successful, long-term exercise club.

Other Requirements

Once you have outlined the goals for your club, you will have to deal with practical matters of location, time, and the type of membership that you wish to attract.

Location. There are several things to consider when you try to find a suitable location for pace walking on a regular basis. The area should be readily accessible, and adequate parking should be nearby. The routes should be of a suitable length for most members, so they can maintain a pace that is comfortable for them. For those members who are concerned with speed or distance, you should measure the exact distance to be covered.

The routes should also be pleasant, reasonably flat, shady in spots, well paved, and have little, if any, traffic. Parks, country lanes, back roads, side streets, and the peripheries of large shopping malls or parking lots are all good places to consider.

Time. Choosing a good time of day and the number of days per week for your pace-walking sessions is an essential part of any plan. You may want to meet once a week (usually on weekends) to exercise together, and members can do their weekday workouts on their own or with other club members on an individual basis. If agreeable, you may all choose to meet regularly during the week.

Some people prefer to work out in the early morning before breakfast. Others choose to exercise in the late afternoon, because working out tends to curb dinnertime appetites. If the club is large enough, you can schedule workouts at both times.

In addition to pace-walking sessions, members may also profit from having a monthly evening meeting, perhaps with a speaker or other activities.

Membership. Many people pace walk—the young, the old, athletes, non-athletes, weight reducers, and those recuperating from an illness. A club is more likely to succeed if it is open to everyone, including those who are unaccustomed to exercising but simply want to try.

But some groups may prefer to concentrate on a particular goal, such as losing weight. In that case, make it clear to potential members and confine eligibility to those who are interested in this specific purpose.

Spreading the Word

Unless you have access to large groups, you will have to publicize the new club to attract potential members. If you have done your homework—established your goals, laid out several suitable routes, and carefully planned your exercise schedule—it's time to investigate your publicity options. For example, you can write up a brief description of the club and its purposes and ask local newspapers to feature it in their community events column. You can also send it to free advertising weeklies.

Another method is to post your notice on every bulletin board you can find, including those at supermarkets, religious centers, social halls, and sporting goods shops. Word of mouth is also a powerful publicizer.

The name of your club can perk up interest, so it's an important factor in your publicity. The words *pace walking* are generic and can be used freely by anyone for any purpose. However, the word *PaceWalkers* is associated with the corporate name PaceWalkers of America, and is protected by a registered trademark.

If you want to use PaceWalkers for the name of your club, contact PaceWalkers of America, Inc. (Box 843, Setauket, NY, 11733; Steven Jonas, M.D., President), to obtain formal authorization for that use. There is no charge for the granting of this permission. However, the word *PaceWalker(s)*® may not be used in print, publicity, promotion, or activities without the permission of PaceWalkers of America, Inc.

How to Initiate a Pace-Walking Contest*

Race walking is a highly technical form of exercising that has strict rules: At least one foot must be in contact with the ground at all times (this distinguishes the sport from running, in which each stride has both feet off the ground for at least an instant), and with each step the knee of the weight-bearing leg must be straight as the body passes over it.

For a variety of reasons, race walks do not attract large numbers of participants. First, it takes some practice and concentration to do the sport correctly. Second, on-the-course judging is required to ensure compliance with the rules, so the organizers of the race walks cannot handle large crowds of participants.

*Based upon "Guide for Creating PaceWalking Contests," an unpublished manuscript originally developed by Dr. Steven Jonas and Gary Westerfield, formerly national women's race walking coach and chairman of the Metropolitan Athletics Congress (N.Y.) Race Walking Committee. It was written in 1990 by Dr. Jonas.

Third, the gait as defined by the rules is not easy to perform except on a flat course, which may be difficult to find. Organized race walks are also traditional races in the sense that the entrants compete to win (although for many that is not the main goal), which may discourage less competitive exercise walkers.

A pace-walking contest provides a different kind of walking competition. Participants race against the clock, not against each other. There is no running—one foot must be in contact with the ground at all times—but there is also no judging. Participants are on the honor system, thus the gait used is entirely up to the individual contestant. And, because the knee can be bent with each step, there is no need to restrict the races to flat courses. The potential number of entrants that can be accommodated in pace-walking contests is limited only by the sophistication of the timing system (see following).

Goals of a Pace-Walking Contest

1. To help provide a focus for health/fitness walking.
2. To promote pace-walking competition at a modest level, without requiring race-walking rules and officiating.
3. To the extent that race-walking organizations sponsor such events, to involve them in the general fitness movement by providing a racing alternative for people who do not want to enter traditional races.
4. To provide a basic level of walking competition that would interest new walkers in race walking.

Rules of a Pace-Walking Contest

Pace walkers compete only against the clock. Every racer who finishes receives an award, such as a ribbon, a button, or a patch. These are differentiated from one another by color, according to the pace maintained during the contest. There are five categories.

1. 18 minutes per mile and over
2. 16:00 to 17:59 minutes per mile
3. 14:00 to 15:59
4. 12:00 to 13:59
5. Under 12 minutes per mile (Cyclists call this kind of event *time-trialing* rather than racing.)

Distances vary, from 1 mile to 5 kilometers (3 miles), or more if feasible, depending upon course characteristics, number of entrants, amount of time available to run the contest, and so forth.

Entrants are timed from the moment the start signal is given. If there is a large number of entrants, consider providing a "wave start" so that each entrant will have the opportunity to achieve his or her best time. (*Wave start* means that the total group of entrants is divided into several subgroups, each of manageable size. The first group starts at the start signal, the second starts one minute later, the third starts two minutes later, and so on. See below for a workable scoring system that uses a wave start.)

Scoring Method

This simple scoring method is based on the honor system. Before the start, a registrar records the names of each entrant in the contest (in alphabetical order to the extent that is feasible, or by race number if numbers are used). Someone with a stopwatch is stationed at the finish line. He or she calls out the finish times as each pace walker crosses the line, and each contestant takes his or her own time in this fashion. (Neither an official race clock nor race numbers are needed, although they could be used if desired.) Then each finisher reports to the person maintaining the list of entrants (the registrar) to have his or her time recorded.

The registrar works out the equivalent minutes-per-mile times for the course beforehand. For example, if the course is 1.3 miles long, the under 12 minutes-per-mile finishers will complete it in less than 15 minutes and 34 seconds (15:34), then 12:00 to 13:59 minutes-per-mile finishers in 15:35 to 18:10, and so forth. (Just multiply the upper and lower ends of each scoring category that you are using by the length of the course, assuming it is more than 1 mile long.) It is then only a matter of handing out the appropriate rewards to each entrant.

For races of up to 50 people, only 2 or 3 race officials are required, primarily the starter/timer and the registrar. It is helpful to have a third person stationed 20 to 30 yards before the finish line to remind entrants to get their times as they cross the line.

Most pace walkers race at a 13 to 15 minutes-per-mile pace. If you are concerned about having a crush of entrants at the end, send the entrants off in waves, as explained previously. First, have people seed (group) themselves by their expected finish time. Then set up your waves so that you have people from each seed in each wave. Start the waves consecutively, 1 minute apart. Thus you will have slow, medium, and fast people going off every minute. The total group of entrants will then spread over the course.

In a wave start race, entrants should be instructed to remember their *actual* finish time as they cross the finish line, not their adjusted time. The adjustment is to be made by the registrar, who will have noted which wave each starter is in and entered that information on the score sheet. Then, as each pace walker reports his or her time, the registrar deducts the correct time allowance.

If you organize a series of contests, you might provide awards for walkers moving up by one or more categories in succeeding contests. A special charge could be made for providing this kind of registration.

Suggested Readings and General References

Suggested Readings

Note: The books and magazines included in this list, unless a Consumer Reports Books publication, are not specifically endorsed by Consumers Union. The reader should also note that recipes in recommended cookbooks, unless they are Consumer Reports Books, have not been tested by Consumers Union.

Cooking

Here is a group of cookbooks from Consumer Reports Books presenting a variety of low-fat recipes.

Cutler, Carol, and the Editors of Consumer Reports Books. *Catch of the Day.* Yonkers, N.Y.: Consumer Reports Books, 1990.

Kaufman, Phyllis C., and the Editors of Consumer Reports Books. *Good Eating, Good Health Cookbook.* Yonkers, N.Y.: Consumer Reports Books, 1990.

Kreitzman, Sue, and the Editors of Consumer Reports Books. *Slim Cuisine.* Yonkers, N.Y.: Consumer Reports Books, 1991.

———, and the Editors of Consumer Reports Books. *Sumptuous Desserts the Slim Cuisine Way.* Yonkers, N.Y.: Consumer Reports Books, 1993.

Scott, Maria Louisa, Jack D. Scott, and the Editors of Consumer Reports Books. *Bean, Pea, and Lentil Cookbook.* Yonkers, N.Y.: Consumer Reports Books, 1991.

The American Heart Association publishes two comprehensive cookbooks for healthy eating.

American Heart Association. *Cookbook.* 5th ed. New York: Times Books/Random House, 1991.

American Heart Association. *Low-Fat, Low-Cholesterol Cookbook.* New York: Times Books/Random House, 1990.

Here are some other low-fat cookbooks that you might want to try.

Oxmoor House. *Light and Easy Cooking Collection.* Birmingham, Ala.: Oxmoor House, 1990.

Piscatella, Joseph C. *Controlling Your Fat Tooth.* New York: Workman Publishing, 1991.

Spear, Ruth. *Low Fat and Loving It.* New York: Warner Books, 1991.

Exercise

Running. These books are oldies but goodies (and still in print as of 1992).

Fixx, Jim. *The Complete Book of Running.* New York: Random House, 1977.

Gallaway's Book on Running. Bolinas, Calif.: Shelter Publications, 1984.

Glover, Bob, and Pete Schuder. *The Competitive Runner's Handbook.* New York: Viking Penguin, 1988.

———, and J. Shepherd. *The Runner's Handbook.* New York: Viking Penguin, 1985.

Recent books include:

Hanc, John. *The Essential Runner.* New York: Lyons and Burford, 1993.

Lebow, Fred, Gloria Averbuch, and friends. *The New York Road Runners Club Complete Book of Running.* New York: NYRRC, 1992.

Bicycling

LeMond, Greg, and K. Gordis. *Greg LeMond's Complete Book of Bicycling.* New York: Perigee/Putnam, 1990.

Lieb, Thom. *Everybody's Book of Bicycle Riding.* Emmaus, Pa.: Rodale Press, 1981.

Swimming and water exercise

Katz, Jane. *Swimming for Total Fitness.* Garden City, N.Y.: Dolphin Books/Doubleday, 1981.

———. *The W.E.T. Workout.* New York: Facts on File, 1985.

Thomas, D. G. *Swimming: Steps to Success.* Champaign, Ill.: Human Kinetics Publishers, 1989.

Walking

Kashiwa, Ann, and James Rippe. *Rockport's Fitness Walking for Women.* New York: Perigee/Putnam, 1987.

Meyers, C. *Walking: A Complete Guide to the Complete Exercise.* New York: Random House, 1992.

Yanker, Gary. *Complete Book of Exercise Walking.* Chicago: Contemporary
   Books, 1983.
   Aerobics
Fox, Molly, and Debra Broide. *Molly Fox's Step On It.* New York: Avon Books,
   1991.
Lance, K. *Low-Impact Aerobics.* New York: Crown Publishers, 1988.
Rosas, D., and C. Rosas, with K. Martin. *Non-Impact Aerobics.* New York: Vil-
   lard, 1987.
   Weight Training
Baechle, T. R., and B. R. Groves. *Weight Training: Steps to Success.* Champaign,
   Ill.: Leisure Press, 1992.
Schwarzenegger, Arnold. *Arnold's Bodybuilding for Men.* New York: Fireside/
   Simon and Schuster, 1981.
Vedral, Joyce. *Now or Never.* New York: Time Warner, 1986.
   Triathloning
Jonas, Steven. *Triathloning for Ordinary Mortals.* New York: W. W. Norton,
   1986.
Tinley, Scott. *Scott Tinley's Winning Triathlon.* New York: Contemporary
   Books, 1986.
   Periodicals
Runner's World. Rodale Press, Emmaus, Pa.
Bicycling. Rodale Press, Emmaus, Pa.
The Walking Magazine. Walking, Inc., Boston, Mass.
Triathlon Today. Ann Arbor, Mich.

References

Introduction

Bennion, Lynn J., Edwin L. Bierman, James M. Ferguson, and the Editors of
   Consumer Reports Books. *Straight Talk About Weight Control.* Yonkers,
   N.Y.: Consumer Reports Books, 1991.
Garner, D. M., and S. C. Wooley. "Confronting the Failure of Behavioral and
   Dietary Treatments for Obesity." *Clinical Psychology Review* 11 (1991):
   729–80.
Jonas, Steven, and Virginia Aronson. *The "I-Don't-Eat (but-I-Can't-Lose)"
   Weight-Loss Program.* New York: Rawson/Macmillan, 1989.

Miller, W. R., and S. Rollnick. *Motivational Interviewing: Preparing People to Change Addictive Behavior.* New York: Guilford Press, 1991.

Schachter, Stanley. "Recidivism and Self-Cure of Smoking and Obesity." *American Psychologist* 37 (1982): 436.

Shaw, Carole. "Statement of Policy." *Big Beautiful Woman* (February 1992): 4.

1 Pathways to Overweight

Bennett, W. I. "Obesity Is Not an Eating Disorder." *Mental Health Letter* 8, no. 4 (October 1991).

Bennion, Lynn J., Edwin L. Bierman, James M. Ferguson, and the Editors of Consumer Reports Books. *Straight Talk About Weight Control.* Yonkers, N.Y.: Consumer Reports Books, 1991.

Berg, F. M. "'Unhappy' Fat Cell Seeks Balance." *Obesity and Health* (March/April 1992): 25.

Bortz, Sharon S. "Not All Calories Are Alike." *Shape* (April 1989): 32.

Brownell, Kelly D. "Weight Control and Physical Exercise." In *Nutrition and Physical Exercise: A Symposium in Observance of National Nutrition Month, Summary of the Proceedings.* Washington: U.S. Department of Health and Human Services, Office of Disease Prevention and Health Promotion, March 28, 1984.

Flatt, J. P. "The Biochemistry of Energy Expenditure." In *Obesity,* edited by P. Bjornstrop and B. N. Brodoff. Philadelphia: n.d.

Hirsch, J., and R. L. Rudolph. "New Light on Obesity." *New England Journal of Medicine* 318 (1988): 509.

———, et al. "The Fat Cell." *Medical Clinics of North America* 73, no. 1 (January 1989): 83.

Katahn, Martin. *The T-Factor Diet.* New York: W. W. Norton, 1989.

Leibel, R. L., et al. "Physiologic Basis for the Control of Body Fat Distribution in Humans." *Annual Review of Nutrition* 9 (1989): 417.

Lissner, L., et al. "Variability of Body Weight and Health Outcomes in the Framingham Population." *New England Journal of Medicine* 324 (1991): 1839.

Mole, P. A., et al. "Exercise Reverses Depressed Resting Metabolic Rate Produced by Severe Caloric Restriction." *Medicine and Science in Sports and Exercise* 21 (1989): 29.

Remington, Dennis, G. Fisher, and E. Parent. *How to Lower Your Fat Thermostat.* Provo, Utah: Vitality House International, 1983.

Shaw, Carole. "Death Rattle of the Diet Decades." *Big Beautiful Woman* (October 1991): 31.

———, with Jane Milstead. "Diets Don't Work!!" *Big Beautiful Woman* (November 1991): 35.

Stern, J. S., and P. Johnson. "Size and Number of Adipocytes and Their Implications." In *Advances in Modern Nutrition: Diabetes, Obesity, and Vascular Disease,* edited by H. M. Katzen and R. J. Mahler. Washington: Hemisphere, 1977.

———, et al. "Obesity: Does Exercise Make a Difference?" In *Recent Advances in Obesity Research,* vol. 5, edited by E. M. Berry et al. London: John Libbey & Co. Ltd., 1987.

Stunkard, Albert J. "Some Perspectives on Human Obesity: Its Causes." *Bulletin of the New York Academy of Medicine* 64 (1988): 902.

Wadden, Thomas A., et al. "Long-term Effects of Dieting on Resting Metabolic Rate in Obese Outpatients." *Journal of the American Medical Association* 264 (1990): 707.

2   *Motivation and Goals*

Bennion, Lynn J., Edwin L. Bierman, James M. Ferguson, and the Editors of Consumer Reports Books. *Straight Talk About Weight Control.* Yonkers, N.Y.: Consumer Reports Books, 1991.

Brownell, Kelly D. "Dieting and the Search for the Perfect Body: Where Physiology and Culture Collide." *Behavior Therapy* 22 (1991): 1–12.

Curry, S. J., and E. H. Wagner. "Evaluation of Intrinsic and Extrinsic Motivation Interventions with a Self-help Smoking Cessation Program." *Journal of Consulting and Clinical Psychology* 59 (1991): 318.

Dwyer, Johanna. "Reducing the Great American Waistline." *American Journal of Public Health* 76 (1986): 1287.

Miller, W. R., and S. Rollnick. *Motivational Interviewing: Preparing People to Change Addictive Behavior.* New York: Guilford Press, 1991.

National Institutes of Health. *Consensus Development Conference Statement: Health Implications of Obesity,* vol. 5, no. 9. Bethesda, Md.: NIH, 1985.

O'Neill, M. "A Growing Movement Fights Diets Instead of Fat." *The New York Times,* 12 April 1992.

Prochaska, James O., and Carlo C. DiClemente. "Transtheoretical Therapy: Toward a More Integrative Model of Change." *Psychotherapy: Theory, Research, and Practice* 19 (1982): 276–88.

Schachter, Stanley. "Recidivism and Self-Cure of Smoking and Obesity." *American Psychologist* 37 (1982): 436.

Shaw, Carole. "Annihilating the Diet Myths." *Big Beautiful Woman* (November 1991): 35.

————. "Realities, Hopes and Dreams: From a BBWoman to Her BBSisters Everywhere." *Big Beautiful Woman* (November 1991): 53.

U.S. Department of Agriculture and U.S. Department of Health and Human Services. *Nutrition and Your Health: Dietary Guidelines for Americans.* 3d ed. Washington: Government Printing Office, 1990.

Webster's New World Dictionary. 2d college ed. New York: World Publishing, 1970.

Williams, L. "Woman's Image in a Mirror: Who Defines What She Sees?" *The New York Times,* 6 February 1992, 1.

3 Pathways to Weight Loss

National Institutes of Health. *Technology Assessment Conference Statement: Methods for Voluntary Weight Loss and Control,* draft. Bethesda, Md.: NIH, revised 1 April 1992.

National Research Council. *Diet and Health.* Washington: National Academy Press, 1989.

Piscatella, Joseph C. *Controlling Your Fat Tooth.* New York: Workman Publishing, 1991.

Salmon, D. M. W., and J. P. Flatt. "Effect of Dietary Fat Content on the Incidence of Obesity Among *Ad Libitum* Fed Mice." *International Journal of Obesity* 9 (1985): 443–49.

U.S. Department of Health and Human Services, Public Health Service. *Surgeon General's Report on Nutrition and Health.* Washington: GPO, 1988. (DHHS [PHS] pub. no. 88–51210).

4 Overweight and You: Self-Assessment

Curry, S. J. and E. H. Wagner. "Evaluation of Intrinsic and Extrinsic Motivation Interventions with a Self-help Smoking Cessation Program." *Journal of Consulting and Clinical Psychology* 59 (1991): 318.

Harvey, A. M., et al. *The Principles and Practice of Medicine.* New York: Appleton-Century-Crofts, 1980.

5 Healthy Eating

American Heart Association. *Diet*. Dallas: AHA, 1985.

————. *Cookbook*. 5th ed. New York: Times Books/Random House, 1991.

American Heart Association. *Nutritious Nibbles*. Dallas: AHA, 1986.

Aronson, Virginia. *Thirty Days to Better Nutrition*. New York: Doubleday, 1984.

Baskin, Rosemary, and the Editors of Consumer Reports Books. *How Many Calories? How Much Fat?* Yonkers, N.Y.: Consumer Reports Books, 1991.

Brownell, Kelly. *The LEARN Program for Weight Control*. Dallas: American Health Publishing, 1991.

Clark, N. "Snack Attack." *The Runner* (January 1987): 20.

Hackman, E. "Eating on the Run." *Runner's World* (July 1987): 61.

Hall, T. "One Who Filled Out on the Low-Fat Fill-Yourself-Up Diet." *New York Times*, 8 January 1992.

Jonas, Steven, and Virginia Aronson. *The "I-Don't-Eat (but-I-Can't-Lose)" Weight-Loss Program*. New York: Rawson/Macmillan, 1989.

Kreitzman, S., and the Editors of Consumer Reports Books. *Slim Cuisine*. Yonkers, N.Y.: Consumer Reports Books, 1991.

National Research Council. *Diet and Health*. Washington: National Academy Press, 1989.

Piscatella, Joseph C. *Controlling Your Fat Tooth*. New York: Workman Publishing, 1991.

Shafquat, S. "Smart Snacking." *Runner's World* (November 1986): 56.

"The Supplement Story: Can Vitamins Help?" *Consumer Reports* (January 1992): 12.

Toufexis, A. "The New Scoop on Vitamins." *Time* (6 April 1992): 54.

University of California at Berkeley. "A Low-fat Diet: 'Pain, but No Gain'?" *Wellness Letter* 8, issue 1 (October 1991): 1.

U.S. Department of Agriculture and U.S. Department of Health and Human Services. *Nutrition and Your Health: Dietary Guidelines for Americans*. 3d ed. Washington: GPO, 1990.

U.S. Department of Health and Human Services, Public Health Service. *Surgeon General's Report on Nutrition and Health*. Washington: GPO, 1988. (DHHS [PHS] pub. no. 88–51210).

6 Healthy Shopping, Healthy Cooking

American Heart Association. *Cookbook*. 5th ed. New York: Times Books/Random House, 1991.

_____. *Low-Fat, Low-Cholesterol Cookbook*. New York: Times Books/Random House, 1990.

Applegate, Liz. "Label-Ease." *Runner's World* (March 1992): 23.

Baskin, Rosemary, and the Editors of Consumer Reports Books. *How Many Calories? How Much Fat?* Yonkers, N.Y.: Consumer Reports Books, 1991.

Burros, Marion. "Eating Well." *The New York Times,* 1 July 1992.

Cutler, C., and the Editors of Consumer Reports Books. *Catch of the Day*. Yonkers, N.Y.: Consumer Reports Books, 1990.

"An End to Label Hype?" *Consumer Reports* (January 1992): 32.

Gasparello, L. "NFPA Files Comments on FDA, USDA Labeling Proposals." *Food and Drink Daily* 2, no. 233 (27 February 1992): 1.

Institute of Medicine. *Nutrition Labeling: Issues and Directions for the 1990s*. Washington: National Academy Press, 1990.

Jonas, Steven, and Virginia Aronson. *The "I-Don't-Eat (but-I-Can't-Lose)" Weight-Loss Program*. New York: Rawson/Macmillan, 1989.

Kaufman, Phyllis C., and the Editors of Consumer Reports Books. *Good Eating, Good Health Cookbook*. Yonkers, N.Y.: Consumer Reports Books, 1990.

Kreitzman, Sue, and the Editors of Consumer Reports Books. *Slim Cuisine*. Yonkers, N.Y.: Consumer Reports Books, 1991.

Mermelstein, N. H. "A Guide to the New Nutrition Labeling Proposals." *Food Technology* (January 1992): 56.

Oxmoor House. *Light and Easy Cooking Collection*. Birmingham, Ala.: Oxmoor House, 1990.

Piscatella, Joseph C. *Controlling Your Fat Tooth*. New York: Workman Publishing, 1991.

Scott, Maria Luisa, and Jack Denton Scott, and the Editors of Consumer Reports Books. *Bean, Pea, and Lentil Cookbook*. Yonkers, N.Y.: Consumer Reports Books, 1991.

Spear, Ruth. *Low Fat and Loving It*. New York: Warner Books, 1991.

Underwood, Greer. *Gourmet Light*. Yonkers, N.Y.: Consumer Reports Books, 1989.

Van Wagner, L. R. "FDA Reviewing Deluge of NLEA Comments." *Food Processing* (April 1992): 8.

Weight Watchers. *Fast & Fabulous Cookbook*. New York: New American Library, 1983.

7 *Exercise*

Bouchard, C., et al, eds. *Exercise, Fitness, and Health.* Champaign, Ill.: Human
Kinetics, 1988.

Brownell, Kelly. "Weight Control and Physical Exercise." *Nutrition and Phys-
ical Exercise: A Symposium in Observance of National Nutrition Month:
Summary of the Proceedings.* Washington: ODPHP, U.S. Department of
Health and Human Services, 28 March 1984.

———. *The LEARN Program for Weight Control.* Dallas: American Health Publishing, 1991.

Flatt, J. P. "Dietary Fat Content, Exercise and Body Composition." In *Obesity:
Dietary Factors and Control,* edited by D. R. Romsos et al. Tokyo: Japan
Scientific Society Press, 1991.

Glover, Bob, and Pete Schuder. *The Competitive Runner's Handbook.* New York:
Penguin, 1983 (and subsequent editions).

Jonas, Steven and Peter Radetsky. *PaceWalking: The Balanced Way to Aerobic
Health.* New York: Crown, 1988.

Piscatella, Joseph C. *Controlling Your Fat Tooth.* New York: Workman Publishing, 1991.

Stamford, B. "Can You Get Fit Playing Racket Sports?" *The Physician and
Sportsmedicine* 14, no. 1 (January 1986): 208.

———. "Exercise Can't Always Counteract Your Diet." *The Physician and
Sportsmedicine* 18, no. 5 (May 1990): 139.

U.S. Department of Health and Human Services, Public Health Service. *Healthy
People 2000.* Washington, D.C.: GPO, 1991. (DHHS pub. no. [PHS] 91–
50213).

U.S. Preventive Services Task Force. *Guide to Clinical Preventive Services: An
Assessment of the Effectiveness of 169 Interventions.* Baltimore: Williams
and Wilkins, 1989.

8 *The Take Control Exercise Plan*

American College of Sports Medicine. *ACSM Fitness Book.* Champaign, Ill.: Leisure Press, 1992.

Jonas, Steven, and Virginia Aronson. *The "I-Don't-Eat (but-I-Can't-Lose)"
Weight-Loss Program.* New York: Rawson/Macmillan, 1989.

———, and Peter Radetsky. *PaceWalking: The Balanced Way to Aerobic Health.*
New York: Crown, 1988.

Walsh, C. *The Bowerman System.* Los Altos, Calif.: Tafnews Press, 1983.

9   The Range of Sports: Technique and Equipment

American College of Sports Medicine. *ACSM Fitness Book*. Champaign, Ill.: Leisure Press, 1992.

Bailey, C. *The New Fit or Fat*. Boston: Houghton Mifflin, 1991.

Fox, Molly, and Debra Broide. *Molly Fox's Step On It*. New York: Avon Books, 1991.

Jonas, Steven, and Virginia Aronson. *The "I-Don't-Eat (but-I-Can't-Lose)" Weight-Loss Program*. New York: Rawson/Macmillan, 1989.

————, and Peter Radetsky. *PaceWalking: The Balanced Way to Aerobic Health*. New York: Crown, 1988.

Katz, Jane. *The W.E.T. Workout*. New York: Facts on File Publications, 1985.

Latella, F. S., and W. Conkling, and the Editors of Consumer Reports Books. *Get in Shape, Stay in Shape*. Yonkers, N.Y.: Consumer Reports Books, 1989.

Sheehan, George. "Running Wild." *The Physician and Sports Medicine* (October 1986).

Appendix A   Risks and Benefits of Obesity and Weight Loss

Bennion, Lynn J., Edwin L. Bierman, James M. Ferguson, and the Editors of Consumer Reports Books. *Straight Talk About Weight Control*. Yonkers, N.Y.: Consumer Reports Books, 1991.

Garner, D. M., and S. C. Wooley. "Confronting the Failure of Behavioral and Dietary Treatments for Obesity." *Clinical Psychology Review* 11 (1991): 729–80.

Jonas, Steven, and Virginia Aronson. *The "I-Don't-Eat (but-I-Can't-Lose)" Weight-Loss Program*. New York: Rawson/Macmillan, 1989.

Lissner, L., et al. "Variability of Body Weight and Health Outcomes in the Framingham Population." *New England Journal of Medicine* 324 (1991): 1839.

National Institutes of Health. *Consensus Development Conference Statement: Health Implications of Obesity*, vol. 5, no. 9. Bethesda, Md.: NIH, 1985.

National Research Council. *Diet and Health: Implications for Reducing Chronic Disease*. Washington: National Academy Press, 1989.

Schachter, S. "Recidivism and Self-Cure of Smoking and Obesity." *American Psychologist* 37 (1982): 436.

Shaw, C. "Statement of Policy." *Big Beautiful Woman* (February 1992): 4.

U.S. Department of Agriculture and U.S. Department of Health and Human Ser-

vices. *Nutrition and Your Health: Dietary Guidelines for Americans.* 3d
ed. Washington: GPO, 1990.

U.S. Department of Health and Human Services, Public Health Service. *Surgeon General's Report on Nutrition and Health.* Washington: GPO, 1988.
(DHHS [PHS] pub. no. 88–50210).

Appendix B   Being Overweight: The Psychosocial Factors

Bennion, Lynn J., Edwin L. Bierman, James M. Ferguson, and the Editors of
Consumer Reports Books. *Straight Talk About Weight Control.* Yonkers,
N.Y.: Consumer Reports Books, 1991.

Brownell, Kelly D. "Dieting and the Search for the Perfect Body: Where Physiology and Culture Collide." *Behavior Therapy* 22 (1991): 1–12.

Curry, S. J., and E. H. Wagner. "Evaluation of Intrinsic and Extrinsic Motivation Interventions with a Self-help Smoking Cessation Program." *Journal of Consulting and Clinical Psychology* 59 (1991): 318.

Dwyer, J. "Reducing the Great American Waistline." *American Journal of Public Health* 76 (1986): 1287.

Garner, D. M., and S. C. Wooley. "Confronting the Failure of Behavioral and
Dietary Treatments for Obesity." *Clinical Psychology Review* 11 (1991):
729–80.

Jonas, Steven, and Virginia Aronson. *The "I-Don't-Eat (but-I-Can't Lose)"
Weight-Loss Program.* New York: Rawson/Macmillan, 1989.

Lissner, L., et al. "Variability of Body Weight and Health Outcomes in the Framingham Population." *New England Journal of Medicine* 324 (1991):
1839.

Miller, W. R., and S. Rollnick. *Motivational Interviewing: Preparing People to
Change Addictive Behavior.* New York: Guilford Press, 1991.

National Institutes of Health. *Consensus Development Conference Statement:
Health Implications of Obesity,* vol. 5, no. 9. Bethesda, Md: NIH, 1985.

National Research Council. *Diet and Health: Implications for Reducing Chronic
Disease.* Washington: National Academy Press, 1989.

Prochaska, James O., and Carlo C. DiClemente. "Transtheoretical Therapy:
Toward a More Integrative Model of Change." *Psychotherapy: Theory,
Research, and Practice* 19 (1982): 276–88.

Schachter, S. "Recidivism and Self-Cure of Smoking and Obesity." *American
Psychologist* 37 (1982): 436.

Shaw, Carole. "Annihilating The Diet Myths." *Big Beautiful Woman* (November 1991): 35.

―――, with J. Milstead. "Attention Doctors and Dieters: Diets Don't Work!!" *Big Beautiful Woman* (November 1991): 35.

―――, with J. Milstead. "Death Rattle of the Diet Decades." *Big Beautiful Woman* (October 1991): 35.

―――. "Realities, Hopes and Dreams: From a BBWoman to Her BBSisters Everywhere." *Big Beautiful Woman* (November 1991): 53.

―――. "Statement of Policy." *Big Beautiful Woman* (February 1992): 4.

Stunkard, A. "Some Perspectives on Human Obesity: Its Causes." *Bulletin of the New York Academy of Medicine* 64 (1988): 902.

U.S. Department of Agriculture and U.S. Department of Health and Human Services. *Nutrition and Your Health: Dietary Guidelines for Americans.* 3d ed. Washington: GPO, 1990.

U.S. Department of Health and Human Services. *Surgeon General's Report on Nutrition and Health.* Washington: GPO, 1988. (DHHS [PHS] pub. no. 88–50210).

Webster's New World Dictionary. 2d college ed. New York: World Publishing, 1970.

Williams, L. "Woman's Image in a Mirror: Who Defines What She Sees?" *The New York Times,* 6 February 1992.

INDEX